THE PSYCHIATRIST AS EXPERT WITNESS

THE
PSYCHIATRIST AS
EXPERT WITNESS

Thomas G. Gutheil, M.D.
Harvard Medical School
Boston, Massachusetts

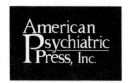

Washington, DC
London, England

Note: The authors have worked to ensure that all information in this book concerning drug dosages, schedules, and routes of administration is accurate as of the time of publication and consistent with standards set by the U.S. Food and Drug Administration and the general medical community. As medical research and practice advance, however, therapeutic standards may change. For this reason and because human and mechanical errors sometimes occur, we recommend that readers follow the advice of a physician who is directly involved in their care or the care of a member of their family.

Copyright © 1998 American Psychiatric Press, Inc.
ALL RIGHTS RESERVED
Manufactured in the United States of America on acid-free paper
First Edition
01 00 99 98   4 3 2

American Psychiatric Press, Inc.
1400 K Street, N.W., Washington, DC   20005
www.appi.org

Library of Congress Cataloging-in-Publication Data
Gutheil, Thomas G.
    The psychiatrist as expert witness / Thomas G. Gutheil.
        p.   cm.
    Companion v. to: The psychiatrist in court.
    Includes bibliographical references and index.
    ISBN 0-88048-763-1 (alk. paper)
    1. Forensic psychiatry—United States.   2. Evidence, Expert—United States.   I. Gutheil, Thomas G.   Psychiatrist in court.
II. Title.
    [DNLM: W 740 G984p 1998]
KF8965.G8   1998
347.73'67—dc21
DNLM/DLC
for Library of Congress   97-29246
                                                                      CIP

British Library Cataloguing in Publication Data
A CIP record is available from the British Library.
Cover image copyright © 1997 PhotoDisc, Inc.

About the Author

Thomas G. Gutheil, M.D., is Professor of Psychiatry at Harvard Medical School, Codirector of the Program in Psychiatry and the Law at the Massachusetts Mental Health Center, and a Fellow of the American Psychiatric Association. He is the first Professor of Psychiatry in the history of Harvard Medical School to be board certified in both general and forensic psychiatry. Through more than 200 publications and international lectures and seminars, he has taught many clinicians about the interfaces between psychiatry and the law. He has received local and national teaching awards, and his textbook *Clinical Handbook of Psychiatry and the Law,* co-authored with Paul S. Appelbaum, M.D., received the Manfred S. Guttmacher Award as the outstanding contribution to forensic psychiatric literature.

To my children and
the hope of the future.
To Shannon,
truly the wind
beneath my wings.

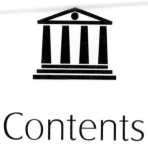

Contents

3

4

5

Discovery and Depositions **59**

6

The Expert in Trial **77**

7

Some Pointers on Expert Witness Practice **97**

8

Writing to and for the Legal System **101**

9

Developing and Marketing a Forensic Practice . . . **111**

10

The Expert on the Road **119**

11

Epilogue 129

APPENDIX 1

Standard Fee Agreement 131

APPENDIX 2

Detailed Fee Agreement 135

APPENDIX 3

Suggested Readings 139

Index 141

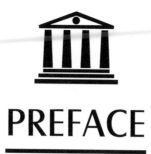

PREFACE

What This Book Is Meant to Do

Serving as an expert witness involves many paradoxes. Such service presents many stresses and equally many satisfactions; it provides tedious stretches of waiting and inactivity interspersed with frenzied bursts of action; it is refreshingly free of managed care and its constraints on good treatment but presents many new and complex restrictions of its own. Often the greatest difficulties in this profession occur at the outset, before experience itself has had the opportunity to provide the most durable and valuable instruction.

This book is targeted to increasing the knowledge and skills of the beginning expert witness and of those contemplating this role for even the first time. Forensic psychiatry is growing in popularity, and many a practitioner feels the urge to dabble a bit in this fascinating realm. This book may provide guidance to you in that activity by drawing on decades of experience in the courtroom and countless beginner's mistakes to help you avoid the same pitfalls.

From another perspective, you might consider this book to be next in chronological order to the companion volume in this series, *The Psychiatrist in Court: A Survival Guide,* which is aimed primarily at the treating psychiatrist who may end up in a courtroom (in fact, if you feel shaky about the basics, that book is a good place to warm up). If your early court experience has not been too traumatic, perhaps—dare I say it—interesting and even fun, you, the novice court goer, may be considering undertaking this activity on a voluntary basis for a change—not being dragged into court, kicking and screaming, but choosing to go. You who are in that position are also my audience.

The more seasoned expert may wish to skim over the more familiar material in the text; for such readers, the later chapters may yet prove useful, in part because they represent material never covered in other sources. Indeed, many an experienced expert has informally lamented to a group of peers how laborious was the early phase of practice when the absence of practical instruction required reinventing the wheel for each new challenge.

This book attempts to provide some of that practical, hands-on mentoring and guidance that were not readily available in the past; whenever possible, concrete advice replaces abstract theorizing, and informal discussion in a user-friendly tone replaces scholarly discourse. I hope you find this approach useful. Best wishes for success in your burgeoning career as an expert witness.

Thomas G. Gutheil, M.D.

Acknowledgments

I am indebted to the Program in Psychiatry and the Law at the Massachusetts Mental Health Center, Harvard Medical School, for the ongoing dialogue and conceptual enrichment that form the underpinning of this work; to Drs. Stephen Behnke, Harold Bursztajn, Larry Strasburger, and Shannon Woolley for their careful review and most helpful critique and comments; and to Ms. Ellen Lewy for absolutely indispensable assistance with the manuscript. The author especially thanks "Dr." James T. Hilliard, Esq., for extremely helpful critique and suggestions and for many years of superb medicolegal advice; Phillip J. Resnick, M.D., for permission to use some of his material on writing for court; and Ms. Candace Love of On-Point Research for valued assistance in compiling resources.

1

Introduction:
What Makes
an Expert?

At first glance, the above question seems to answer itself: expertise makes the expert, that is, knowing a lot about a certain topic and having extensive experience therein.

In the courtroom setting, the question of what makes an expert witness is more complex. A reductionistic answer is this: an expert is anyone whom a court accepts or whom it stipulates as an expert. This is true in the legal sense at a certain level but insufficiently illuminating for the purposes of this book.

In this book, the concept of expert witness, clinically defined, is a psychiatrist who uses particular skills, both clinical and nonclinical, to provide information and understanding relevant to the legal system's concerns. This essentially didactic functioning—more closely resembling teaching than anything else—often requires intellectually bridging the gap between two widely divergent realms of discourse and thought: psychiatry and law. Indeed, this intellectual challenge is one of the features that makes forensic work so exciting and interesting to its practitioners.

Scholars in forensics point to the need for expert witnesses in a primarily educational context; that is, the expert is to educate the attorney, then the judge or jury, about matters that are beyond lay knowledge or decision making. A lay juror is assumed to be capable of deciding which of two contradictory pieces of testimony is more credible. Indeed, it could be argued that this is the essential function of the jury system: a social mechanism to decide which side of a case is to be believed. For that matter, because what an expert offers is "only" a witness's opinion, not the ultimate finding that a judge or jury decides, the jury is free to accept or reject the expert's testimony in whole or in part.

However, some questions can only be answered by a specialist, such as: Did a particular course of treatment meet the medical "standard of care?" Because jurors are not expected to be physicians, the expert must supply the relevant reasoning to permit the jury first to grasp the issue and then to perform its decision-making function.

Under this model, the court system needs expert witnesses in a burgeoning variety of technical fields, from ballistics to the temperature of coffee sold at fast-food franchises. What I find bemusing is the fact that attorneys appearing in public fora such as television shows commonly and disingenuously downplay the need for experts, proclaiming their ultimate faith in the jurors themselves. At times, the attorneys thus pontificating are the same ones who had retained me on a previous case.

A leading plaintiffs' attorney described his need for an expert in this way during a lecture:

> What I think you want the jury to feel when you have an expert in front of them is: "Gee, if I had this problem, I'd want to be treated by this person because he/she makes sense; I believe this person." You want someone who will present in a way that the jurors would

be inclined to say this. I also want someone who has clinical experience and is doing that which he/she is testifying about. . . . I do not
want someone who [merely] teaches others about it.

Another scholar, a law professor, went even further by listing
the functions of the expert as being to 1) tell the story, 2) make the
fact finder want you to win, 3) make sense out of the law, 4) help
the fact finder see the facts, and 5) argue the case (1).

Other scholars suggest that one of the principal functions of the
expert is to tell the story, to draw causal connections between apparently unrelated facts to demonstrate and illuminate the meaning of what has happened. The expert also will show how
conclusions are based on facts in the case as they may relate to
symptoms, demographics, statistics, syndromes, clinical entities,
causation, and the resulting probabilities.

A vivid example of the vital importance of storytelling (from the
lawyer's viewpoint) occurred in one of my first suicide malpractice
cases. The highly experienced defense attorney who had retained
me was heard to mutter at one point, "Where are the communion
pictures?" Pressed for a less cryptic expression, he noted that the
plaintiff's attorney had failed in a crucial storytelling function to
make the person who had committed suicide come alive in the
minds of the jury so that they would be sensitive to what had been
lost by his death. Showing pictures of the deceased at communion, at family functions, and so forth would have accomplished
this vital storytelling purpose.

In this chapter, and throughout this book, I assume some rudi-
mentary familiarity with the courtroom itself and with basic legal
concepts; however, some points, although basic, are so essential
to this work that I review them in the following discussions.

The Adversarial Context

Most clinical work occurs in the context of the alliance; opposition-
ality, conflict between the parties, or an adversarial atmosphere are
problems to be avoided, surmounted, or resolved or otherwise put

to therapeutic use. In medicolegal work, the adversarial context is one of the "givens" in the situation. The beginning expert must take pains to be clear on how this overarching consideration affects the work being done.

The Prime Question

Any forensic psychiatrist, whether testifying or consulting, must first ask the question, for whom am I working? Your answer will clarify your location within the adversarial framework, as well as the usual lack of a physician-patient relationship (that is, in the clinical context, you usually work for the patient; in a forensic setting, you usually do not). Like other consultants, you work for the consultee (that is, in the forensic setting, the retaining attorney). You also will be sensitized to certain issues of privileged information and work product exclusion (a term clarified later in this discussion) that may come to bear. The question of whom you work for also will alert you to major pitfalls of bias, challenging you to maintain your objectivity when your review leads to conclusions unfavorable to the side retaining you.

Note for completeness that certain forensic contexts, such as child custody evaluations, render highly complex the question of agency. The usual guiding principle in such determinations is "the best interests of the child," a mandate that may trump other claims on your agency. This specialized topic is beyond the scope of this book, but experts in child custody issues often stress the value of working directly for the judge as court-appointed evaluator, because that position confers greater neutrality and protection for your efforts.

To clarify the term *work product,* notes, memoranda, files, and other papers that the attorney generates in the course of litigation are called work product, meaning that they are about the case but are not *of* the case. In other words, they are not case-related documents and therefore are protected from disclosure. Communications from the retaining attorney to the expert are generally discoverable, with some exceptions. Most attorneys know not to include details of their trial strategy in letters to you. The retaining attorney will guide you in this matter; when in doubt, your personal attorney can always give you advice on nondiscoverable matters.

Confidentiality Warnings

One of the immediate issues to confront the expert is the fact that therapy, with exceptions, is private and confidential. In contrast, court-related issues are often matters of public record and public exposure (in open court). Therefore, we must pay scrupulous attention to warning the people whom we interview and examine—plaintiffs, defendants, suspects, convicts, litigants, and parties of whatever stripe—that they are not to expect business as usual (meaning usual confidentiality) just because they are talking to a psychiatrist. The warning about the nonconfidentiality of the material to be discussed represents an essential ethical threshold for all forensic work; it should, of course, be carefully documented.

The Database

The term *database* is my own shorthand label for all the relevant materials I may read in the course of a case, including records, legal documents, reports, correspondence, my own or others' interview notes, and relevant literature. The term also suggests that your opinion rests on a base, or basis, of data—facts and clinical verities—rather than on idiosyncratic theory or your whim, fantasy, or impression. Although therapy usually transpires within the patient's self-reported data, the forensic perspective almost always extends beyond the individual examinee. One trenchant reason for this approach is to obtain corroboration or discorroboration.

Malingering and Self-Serving Motivation

Unlike the treatment context, the forensic arena provides a variety of incentives for malingering and self-serving behavior or testimony. It is usually inappropriate for a treating therapist to be suspicious of a patient's truthfulness, absent clear delusions, obvious self-contradiction, and similar signs. In contrast, the forensic practitioner is wise to suspect everyone of having some stake in the matter, be it moral or monetary, and to maintain an appropriately skeptical posture, always seeking out verification, corroboration, or discorroboration for all important facts.

Reasonable Medical Certainty

The investigative efforts previously implied permit the expert to offer testimony at the requisite standard of proof called *reasonable medical certainty* (sometimes described as reasonable psychiatric certainty, reasonable medical probability, or even reasonable psychological certainty). This term does not mean absolute certainty (100% sure) or an impression (1% to 50% sure). Rather, it most often means that the expert is sworn to testify about opinions that are true "more likely than not" or that are 51% certain. Note that there may be some jurisdictional variation on this point; ask about the local variant. Deciding where this level of certainty lies for the expert is one of the critical tasks of forensic work.

The Hired Gun Problem

The so-called hired gun problem continues to dog the field of expert forensic work, makes forensic psychiatrists unpopular with their clinical colleagues, and leads physicians of all specialties, observing, for example, high-profile insanity cases, to declare forensic psychiatry an embarrassment to the field of medicine in general and psychiatry in particular.

The most succinct definition of a hired gun is an expert witness who sells testimony instead of time. All psychiatrists, including forensic psychiatrists, sell *time;* we are paid by time criteria. The hired gun goes beyond time criteria to demonstrate corrupt willingness to offer for money the testimony that the retaining attorney desires, regardless of its clinical validity. Such individuals can be recognized not only by the baselessness of their opinions but also often by their use of 1-800 telephone numbers. Although there are exceptions, a number of experts point out that no honest witness does enough forensic business to merit a 1-800 telephone number. For most of us, forensic work is a sideline to our clinical focus.

Other contextual clues about the hired gun are overly candid advertising in legal media (for example, "opinions for sale!") and use of expert witness brokerage organizations that specialize in matching willing experts with attorneys. As a general rule, honest experts should avoid these approaches to finding work, if only to avoid guilt by association and possible caricature by opposing attorneys (see also Chapter 9 in this volume).

The importance of having a salaried job or a private clinical practice cannot be overemphasized because these provide a base of financial stability that enables you to turn down cases. If a clearly meritless case is offered to you for review, you must be free to turn it down without feeling that you are kissing good-bye your children's college careers. Thus, you avoid temptation to skew your opinion, and you maintain your ethical compass direction.

There are complexities that should be addressed. Experts who make the mistake of becoming emotionally caught up in their own opinions (instead of recognizing that experienced, ethical experts can disagree) may view anyone's opinion that opposes their own as hired gun material. Often no absolute standard exists by which to measure opinion testimony, so this question may be difficult to resolve in any objective sense without analysis of that expert's database, reasoning, case materials, and corroborating data.

A valuable development in this area has been the introduction of peer review for testimony as a voluntary educational aid provided by the American Academy of Psychiatry and the Law (AAPL).

Experts concerned about their testimony in conflict with a peer's opinion may submit that testimony to the AAPL Peer Review Committee for consideration. Forensic psychiatrists who have made use of this committee find it extremely helpful and illuminating. (By the way, all forensic psychiatrists should seriously consider joining the AAPL and attending its meetings; it is an excellent way to benefit from the teaching of colleagues and to share ideas.)

The Humility Factor

Finally, it is always worth keeping in mind the sobering fact that the expert's contribution may not be all that determinative of case outcome. Early in my career, I bid farewell to the fantasy that I would "win" the case by profound scholarship and dazzling testimony on the stand. Some attorneys report that their only use of experts is to neutralize or cancel out the testimony (or even the mere presence) of the experts on the other side, thus leaving the jury free to vote its "gut." Even when the expert is the only source of data that the jury receives, it is often the case that the outcome of the legal matter has been predetermined entirely by the selection of the jury before the trial even starts.

The issues outlined throughout this chapter should be kept in mind while reading the remainder of this book.

Reference

1. Dragan EF: Creative use of experts: what is an expert used for? Council for the Advancement of Science in Law, Expert's Quarterly, Winter 1997, p 2

Suggested Readings

Ackerman MJ, Kane AW: Psychological Experts in Divorce, Personal Injury and Other Civil Actions. New York, Wiley, 1993

Appelbaum PS: The role of the mental health professional in court. Hosp Community Psychiatry 36:1043–1046, 1985

Appelbaum PS: Forensic psychiatry: the need for self-regulation. Bull Am Acad Psychiatry Law 20:153–162, 1992

Bronstein DA: Law for the Expert Witness. Boca Raton, FL, Lewis Publishers, 1993

Diamond BL: The forensic psychiatrist: consultant versus activist in legal doctrine. Bull Am Acad Psychiatry Law 2:119–132, 1992

Dietz PE: The forensic psychiatrist of the future. Bull Am Acad Psychiatry Law 15:217–227, 1987

Golding SL: Mental health professionals and the courts: the ethics of expertise. Int J Law Psychiatry 13:281–307, 1990

Gutheil TG, Rachlin S, Mills MJ: Differing conceptual models in psychiatry and law, in Legal Encroachment on Psychiatric Practice. Edited by Rachlin S. San Francisco, CA, Jossey-Bass, 1985, pp 5–11

Miller JA: The psychiatrist as expert witness, in Expert Witness. Edited by Rossi FF. Chicago, IL, American Bar Association, 1991, pp 509–528

Quen JM: The psychiatrist as expert witness, in The Psychiatrist in the Courtroom. Edited by Quen JM. Hillsdale, NJ, Analytic Press, 1994, pp 233–248

Smith SR: Mental health expert witnesses: of science and crystal balls. Behavioral Sciences and the Law 7:145–180, 1989

2

The Expert's Ethical Universe

My first adventure in the witness chair convinced me that it was as unstable as a one-wheeled rickshaw on a downhill course, with two steering controls manned by lawyers intent upon veering the contraption in opposite directions at every fork in the road, while a judge alternately stomped on an unreliable accelerator and an unpredictable brake . . . [Finally] I realized that each witness chair comes equipped with a stabilizer control. It is a control easily within the reach of every witness—the lever marked "truth." (1, p. S-3)

The expert faces many challenges in forensic work, but the one that often poses the greatest challenge is maintaining your ethical bearings against the manifold pressures that attempt to lead you astray. In this chapter, I address these ethical concerns and the means by which to keep your internal compass pointing to "ethical north."

The Nonconfidentiality Warning

Although nonconfidentiality has been broached in Chapter 1 in this volume, it is so central to the forensic relationship as opposed to the clinical one that it bears repeating for several reasons. First, examinees being interviewed by a psychiatrist, particularly an empathically attuned one, tend to drift unconsciously into a "therapeutic mode." They may forget that this encounter is *not* therapy, and its results may harm, rather than help, their ultimate goals in the legal process. To prevent such inadvertent abuse or exploitation of the examinee, the ethical expert begins with warnings about the differences between the forensic and clinical interview and, if necessary, repeats those warnings if the examinee appears to be slipping into a state of therapeutic self-disclosure. The warnings (carefully documented, of course) are especially important in capital criminal cases in which a life may literally hang in the balance.

Turndown Rates

An ethical test for the expert occurring early in the process is the case turndown rate. This term does not refer to those cases for which you simply do not have sufficient time or those for which there is some conflict (for example, you are friends with one of the defendants). Rather, the turndown rate is the percentage of cases in which, *after* reviewing, you decide you cannot support the retaining attorney's position. (Note that even if you cannot support all of the claims proffered in the case, your attorney still may use your opinion or report to bolster one aspect of the case or to limit the extravagant claims of the expert on the other side.)

For example, in a psychiatric malpractice case for which you have been retained by the plaintiff, your review of the database may lead you to the conclusion that the treaters all practiced within the standard of care. Therefore, this case might be called a defense case because the actions of the defendants are, indeed, defensible. You pass this information on to your retaining attorney, who—in the ideal situation—accepts this view, thanks you for your help, indicates the intention of explaining your information to the client, and states, understandably, that the firm will not be using you as an expert. After settling up any monetary adjustments, this case is over and has been turned down.

For completeness, note that in the not-so-ideal situation, the attorney curses your name, denounces your integrity, impugns your ancestors, scoffs at your qualifications, and slams down the telephone. This fortunately rare emotional response is a powerful argument for obtaining a retainer in advance.

Most experts find it helpful to note what percentage of the time they turn a case down as an ethical orienting device. Turndown rates between 10% and 30% are not uncommon. If you take every case you review, you must consider whether your threshold for case validity may be too low. If you turn down most cases you get, either your threshold for validity is too high or you need to meet a better class of attorneys.

For symmetry, it is also valuable to scrutinize the flip side of this issue: how often do you give the retaining attorney exactly what he or she wants?

Note also that you may be in a position to refer cases to colleagues who are known to you as having perspectives different from your own on, for example, inpatient care. Although these referrals are not strictly turndowns, they do represent cases in which you have elected not to participate.

The turndown decision is often difficult to evaluate because you have no control over the kind of cases referred to you, only over those you elect to accept. Consequently, you could receive a number of good cases, all of which you might accept, or a number of invalid or meritless cases, all of which you should turn down. Nevertheless, it is worthwhile keeping mental or written track of the number of cases you turn down and the percentage of the total as a kind of ethical filter.

Ethics and the Oath

Taking the oath at deposition or trial is another ethical threshold. You are agreeing from that point on to offer only that testimony that you can swear to rather than what you think, guess, speculate about, and so on.

An author described the special sensitivity to what one can swear to in this way: You are asked, "What color is that house over there?" The novice answers, "White." Your correct answer would be, "White on this side." Once under oath, that is, you take nothing for granted.

Scholars in forensics have discussed two models of apparent equal integrity concerning the practical meaning of taking the oath (2). One model holds that once the oath is taken, the only touchstone is absolute truth as you know it or understand it. Partisan pressures from the adversary are put aside, and the expert becomes the fully neutral observer and reporter. This model is sometimes called the *advocate for truth model.*

The second model holds that accepting the reality of the adversarial system is simply part of being an expert because that is the arena in which you work. Consequently, it is fully acceptable to advocate for the side that retained you by testifying as effectively and persuasively as you are able, as long as 1) you are frank about the limits of your data (including contrary data) and therefore of your testimony, and 2) you answer cross-examination truthfully (see the following discussion). This model has been called the *honest advocate model.* Advocacy for your opinion is always acceptable.

In forensic practice, most experts use a combination of these models as a means of arriving at the critical ethical posture of "honest expert."

Problems of Loyalty and Identification

The relationship between the expert and the retaining attorney may undergo the vicissitudes of other professional alliances, but two dimensions of the relationship pose potential ethical problems.

First, under the rubric of loyalty, just what does the expert owe the retaining attorney? Strictly speaking, you owe only serious, committed quality work; you do not owe agreement with the attorney's position or theory of the case. The novice expert who adjusts or bends or twists an opinion away from clinically based validity, out of feelings of being loyal to his or her retaining attorney, is misreading the nature of the ethical contract between the two parties.

I suggest you also owe rigorous candor to your retaining attorney about what you can and cannot say and what the weaknesses in your own opinion are. The worst betrayal of the attorney-expert contract is the shock and surprise that an attorney feels when your testimony in deposition or on the stand takes a turn totally out of synchrony with your previous disclosures and discussions with the attorney. You do owe it to your attorney to level with him or her about yourself (for example, the skeletons in your closet, discussed further in Chapter 3 in this volume), your opinion and its limitations, and what you can and cannot testify to under oath. If the attorney, with whom you have done many a previous case together, is disappointed that your present opinion is unfavorable, that is not your problem. The attorney is free to find another expert, settle or drop the case, or make whatever use of your opinion that may be of service.

A pitfall in this area might be called forensic countertransference, that is, identification with your retaining attorney. As you work closely with your attorney, you may come to like, respect, and admire him or her. These quite natural feelings may yet lead to an identification with the attorney and with the attorney's goals; this identification may compromise your needed objectivity. Recall that the attorney's goals are winning the case; yours are providing ethical and valid consultation or testimony or both. This difference is significant.

Extending this idea, might extensive socializing with the retaining attorney—or, similarly, being retained by an attorney with whom you have had an extensive previous social relationship —constitute a problem? The answer probably depends on the maturity of both parties, but the likelihood of identification bias would surely seem to be greater; thus, this factor would require greater scrutiny of the relationship by the forensic witness.

Note for completeness that the partisan effect of loyalty to the attorney is significantly bypassed when you serve as a court-appointed expert or examiner. This neutral position is highly desirable for that reason, although not common in practice. The fact that the position is more or less neutral does not, of course, eliminate other subtler biasing factors, such as overidentification with the judge or the "system."

Note also that, as a clinician, you are expected to manage your countertransference toward the examinee or the examinee's actions; if the countertransference is unmanageable, you should refer the case. If you are a victim of child molestation, for instance, you may feel unable to examine objectively a child molester. There is no shame in this.

The Ultimate Ethical Test

The ultimate test of expert witness integrity is honesty under cross-examination. On direct examination, the lawyer will take you through your credentials, what you have reviewed, your opinion, and its basis. A competent attorney and expert will have prepared for this stage of the proceedings by reviewing the questions that the attorney plans to ask, clearing up any dubious issues, anticipating relevant cross-examination, and so on.

Cross-examination is new territory, spontaneous and unrehearsed. During the cross-examination, the holes and limits of your side of this case will likely be explored. Therefore, your ultimate test as an expert is your honesty under cross-examination when you must acknowledge, if appropriately asked by the other side, the limits of your credentials, the limits of your data, the limits of your knowledge, the limits of your conclusions, and the limits of your testimony.

In the process of cross-examination, experts can be separated into two categories. The less admirable experts, having become inappropriately enamored of their opinions rather than of the truth, defend those opinions passionately and fiercely on cross-examination, and their testimony is often unconvincing. The more admirable experts calmly acknowledge the details of the case unfavorable to their opinion, the true extent of their opinions, and the hypothetical situations under which their conclusions would be different. Such candor may well enhance their credibility. Again, none of this information should be a surprise to your attorney.

References

1. Baker TO: Operator's Manual for a Witness Chair. Milwaukee, WI, Defense Research Institute, 1983
2. Appelbaum PS, Gutheil TG: Clinical Handbook of Psychiatry and the Law, 2nd Edition. Baltimore, MD, Williams & Wilkins, 1991

Suggested Readings

Appelbaum PS: Psychiatric ethics in the courtroom. Bull Am Acad Psychiatry Law 12:225–231, 1984

Appelbaum PS: In the wake of Ake: the ethics of expert testimony in an advocate's world. Bull Am Acad Psychiatry Law 15:15–25, 1987

Appelbaum PS: The parable of the forensic psychiatrist: ethics and the problem of doing harm. Int J Law Psychiatry 13:249–259, 1990

Hollien H: The expert witness: ethics and responsibilities. J Forensic Sci 35:1414–1423, 1990

Katz J: The fallacy of the impartial expert. Bull Am Acad Psychiatry Law 20:141–152, 1992

Miller RD: Professional vs personal ethics: methods for system reform. Bull Am Acad Psychiatry Law 20:163–177, 1992

Rogers R: Ethical dilemmas in forensic evaluations. Behavioral Sciences and the Law 5:149–160, 1987

Schultz-Ross RA: Ethics and the expert witness. Hosp Community Psychiatry 44:388–389, 1993

Weinstock R: Perceptions of ethical problems by forensic psychiatrists. Bull Am Acad Psychiatry Law 17:189–202, 1989

Weinstock R, Leong GG, Silva JA: Opinions by AAPL forensic psychiatrists on controversial ethical guidelines: a survey. Bull Am Acad Psychiatry Law 19:237–248, 1991

3

First Principles

In clinical work, the patient is your employer; that is usually clear. In the forensic relationship, your employer is less clear. As noted in Chapter 2 in this volume, forensic work should thus always begin with the question, for whom am I working? This orienting query about "agency" dictates to whom certain duties lie and how priorities should be set. When you examine a plaintiff at a defense attorney's request, you may—indeed, you should—be polite and supportive to your examinee, but you are not required to preview your findings, make recommendations, prescribe, treat, or perform some other such intervention with him or her. Your duty is to the person for whom you are working; that person is the recipient of your opinions. That relationship is also a source of certain pitfalls of bias, discussed later in this chapter. Consultative experience suggests that the failure to ask the basic question of agency is the frequent cause of inadequate examination, ineffectual testimony, and compromised working relationship.

Although you are usually working for an attorney, you may or may not owe a separate allegiance to that attorney's client. However, you certainly do not owe a duty to other professionals who may be part of your examinee's treatment team, as when a defendant, considered for examination of competence to stand trial, is being treated in a hospital setting.

If you are examining one of a group of plaintiffs or defendants with separate representation (such as a tort case concerning toxins, or some kind of class action), you still work only for your attorney and your attorney's client, regardless of what is going on with other experts or treaters.

The issue of not serving as expert when you are the treater is relevant but is extensively discussed in the companion volume, *The Psychiatrist in Court: A Survival Guide,* and in Appendix 1 to that volume. If this issue is in question, refer to those sources.

Initial Negotiations With the Retaining Attorney

Although psychotherapy is generally said to begin at the moment of eye contact between patient and therapist, an expert witness relationship usually begins with a telephone conversation between you and the attorney who is seeking an expert. This telephone call is far from a mere administrative formality. Instead, some vital information must be obtained to make the entire future relationship smoother and more valuable to both parties. In this chapter, the term *your attorney* will be used to refer to the attorney retaining you as an expert, not your personal counsel.

How you communicate with your attorney is important from the outset. Novice experts sometimes believe that their goal in the first telephone call from the attorney is to impress the latter with their erudition, clinical experience, and mastery of professional jargon; this approach is self-defeating. Attorneys are looking for a psychiatrist who can communicate clearly and simply with them and lay juries. Friendly, informal discussion should be the format; politeness dictates that you call the attorney Mr. or Ms. Smith until he or she invites you to call him or her John or Jane.

The following discussions include queries about issues that the expert should contemplate before agreeing to consult on the case.

The Retaining Attorney's Request

What exactly am I being asked to do as a psychiatrist? What are the clinical and forensic issues? Are they rational? Are these issues that a psychiatrist actually has some knowledge about; that is, what is the psychiatric aspect of this case? A certain percentage of cases will turn out to be ones in which your role is presumed to be that of human lie detector, as though by a simple examination of the plaintiff you can supposedly determine the truth of the claim. In general, such cases should be reality-tested for the attorney.

Your Fitness as an Expert

Should you, personally, take on this case? Do you have some expertise in this general area or in this specific area? If you do not, but the attorney wishes to retain you anyway because of a recommendation from a peer or because of the high regard in which you are held by local physicians, it becomes your responsibility to be completely candid about the limitations of your knowledge and experience (for example, "Look, I don't know a great deal about this specific subject, but I am willing to become familiar with the issue."). The attorney can then take or leave this arrangement. Note that your special expertise should exist against a backdrop of your general competence in the field, as indicated by publication, experience, board certification, and so on.

The Question of Bias

Is there an element of bias pro or con? Do you know the players, the hospital, and the setting? Are there personal resonances with the case that would interfere with your objectivity? For example, if your aged mother has just died in a nursing home, you should probably consider turning down an emotional injury case involving an elderly female nursing home resident. This example is fairly obvious, but subtler versions of personal resonance with a case are not uncommon.

These issues go beyond mere conflict of interest, which is usually (but not always) clear-cut. I recommend hearing about the broad issues of the case first and only then asking for people's names. Therefore, if you cannot or should not take the case, the attorney will not have revealed confidential information to you (the names), yet you will have screened for bias before the attorney has taken you too deeply into trial strategy issues that should be kept privileged and private.

The Expert's History as Possible Problem Area

Are there any blots on your reputation? Your attorney is entitled to know whether any circumstances could prove embarrassing if brought up by the other side in court. For example, have you been the defendant in a malpractice suit, however baseless? Are you now being investigated by the board of registration for some allegation, no matter how unfounded? Do you have a history of problems in the military, juvenile offenses, a criminal record (no matter how minor), credentialing problems in the past, and similar problems? You must be extremely candid with the lawyers about such facts at the outset.

Are things you have written a problem for this particular case? Attorneys hate being surprised by the fact that an article you wrote 5 years earlier, for instance, contradicts your present position, even if the issues are clinically totally different. Do your best to address this possibility early. Reviewing your own published work in a particular area is a worthwhile part of your preparation. If you write a lot, you realize that the more you write, the more words you might have to eat on cross-examination.

Similarly, are there cases in which you have testified on behalf of the other side, have taken an opposite position or opinion, or have been retained by one side more than the other? Review this with the attorney. Vast amounts of deposition and trial testimony are now stored on mainframe computers and thus are available to any attorney who searches for it.

Time, Fees, and Other Embarrassments

A judge in a recent case had this to say about experts:

> It has been the experience and observation of this court that in all the medical malpractice trials over which it has presided, the ultimate beneficiaries, in an economic sense, are truly the physicians who demand and usually obtain exorbitant compensation for their testimony [sic] as expert witnesses. . . . In too many medical malpractice cases, unfortunately, the Hippocratic Oath has been supplanted by opportunism and greed by those who participate as medical expert witnesses. (1)

This quote is interesting from several viewpoints. As is often the case, attorneys are invisible within the court record; for example, the court record chidingly notes, "Smith failed to plead . . . " when everyone, including the speaker, knows that it was Smith's *lawyer* who was derelict. Thus, in the preceding quote, the judge elects to be blind to the legal opportunism paraded before him daily— attorneys have been known to look for an occasional monetary incentive in bringing particular cases forward—and instead focuses on the experts, who are the strangers in the courtroom.

Second, the judge commits the technical error that yet captures perfectly the public perception: the experts are being paid for their *testimony* (that is, they are all corrupt), not for their time and clinical expertise. This issue is further discussed later in this chapter.

Like the judge previously quoted, opposing attorneys enjoy labeling the opposing expert as a hired gun (a problem discussed in more detail later in this chapter). Indeed, one of the oldest chestnuts of cross-examining the expert is the familiar "How much are you being paid for your testimony, Doctor?" The only appropriate answer, ideally delivered in a calm tone of voice and not through clenched teeth, is "I am not being paid for my testimony, only for my time." Other witnesses may take this further: "My testimony is not for sale," or "I am paid by the hour, same as you," or "Nothing" (and wait for the attorney to crack, "So, Doctor, this is a pro bono case for you?"). I personally am not convinced that these flourishes add anything to the basic statement above and may sound pompous unless perfectly delivered.

But what makes this subject more than usually difficult is the fact that clinicians already have emotional conflicts about the issue of money, whether for psychotherapy or expert witness time. Therapists who are quite capable of taking an extensive, probing sexual history without a qualm begin to blush and stammer when it comes to discussing money. Several approaches can be used to deal with this conflict beyond simple self-awareness and a thorough personal analysis.

First, choose a fee that you would not be embarrassed to state. Check with your peers at similar levels of training and experience to determine what is customary for your area and be ready to say as much. Second, charge fairly: get a sense of how much time it takes to read forensic material (preferably in a quiet setting, without children bursting in to share their Nintendo triumphs with you), and try to maintain that rate. Use timers or check your watch at the start and end of a piece of work and write down the time. Note also that time spent thinking, planning, analyzing, and organizing your forensic assessment is part of the work.

I also recommend not "nickel and diming." Yes, I know, attorneys have timers on all their phones and charge by the split second, but you are made of finer stuff. Don't charge for a 90-second telephone call confirming the date of a deposition, for instance, or for reading a one-paragraph letter. Then, when asked about your fees on the stand, you can calmly state them without guilt, shame, or other conflict. Urge your attorney to bring up your fees on direct examination to get it out of the way.

How much work or time should you devote to the case? This depends on your schedule. Keep your vacations in mind, and give the dates to the attorney. If you don't have enough time, don't take on the case; it is unfair to your attorney. Beware of taking on so many cases so that you do not have sufficient time and attention to pay to each one.

Bitter experience teaches that it is critically important to have a standard fee agreement or contract signed by the attorney (or insurer) and to operate by retainer or payment in advance. Owen Marshall, Perry Mason, the good folks on "L.A. Law"—these paragons would never *think* of failing to pay an expert's legitimate expenses, but in my experience, failure to pay is reality.

Many experts starting out in the forensic field do not bother with fee agreements until they are "stiffed" by their first attorney. To novice experts, it comes as a surprise that it is *not* an ethical violation for an attorney to stiff his or her expert for a legitimate fee if there is nothing in writing (and in some cases, even if there is). I took my first major "stiffer" to court eventually and received some of my money; in addition, I reported him to the Massachusetts Board of Bar Overseers, the organization in charge of ethical issues, among others. That august body opined that this was not an ethical problem but a business issue or a contract issue. Standard and detailed fee agreements are supplied in Appendixes 1 and 2, respectively, at the end of this book; when you design your own, you will discover that every subordinate clause in each new version will be poured out in blood from your previous failure to anticipate duplicity by some attorney.

Ethically speaking, your fee should never be contingent; you are charging for time regardless of the outcome of the case. The attorneys, of course, are free to employ contingent fees, but your consultation must be free of investment in any form in the outcome of the case. It should, ideally, be a matter of indifference to you who wins a case. You give only testimony. You sell only time. Refuse any other arrangement.

Roles of the Expert

What exactly will be your role in the case at hand? Experts may be retained for a range of legitimate, basically consultative services, some of which never lead to the courtroom. You simply may be a consultant to the attorney on the merits of the case at the outset. You may be needed to evaluate a plaintiff (or a defendant, for that matter). You may consult to the attorney on matters of clinical reasoning to determine whether the complaint makes clinical sense. You might advise the attorney on how to cross-examine the other side's experts or litigants. You may provide rebuttal material for use by others. You may play some combination of the foregoing roles or all of these roles and then serve as expert witness in the courtroom.

Will you be expected to testify at trial, or is the matter likely not to go to trial? Are you going to be a reporter, that is, someone who has to generate a written report, or will your opinion be used by the attorney to strategize without a report, which might have to be supplied to the other side? All these considerations affect not only your clear sense of role but also practical matters such as your time allotment and scheduling. If you are, at some point, going to testify, is a tentative trial date known? How do your vacations fit in? This information allows you to allot more time and spread your cases so that you are not testifying on consecutive days for different cases—the expert's nightmare.

The Final Decision

Putting together everything that you now know—what you charge, what your time permits, what your skills or knowledge support, how you feel about the attorney, how free from bias or conflict the situation is—finally ask, should you take the case or should you turn it down?

The above sequence of queries is part of a negotiating process between you and the attorney or the law firm or even, rarely, an individual client. As a rule, working for the attorney or insurer is a better idea than working for the client alone. Among other things, your consultative, nontreatment role is clearer. Moreover, your attorney, as a professional, is more accountable.

The Stage of Case Review

Let us assume you have agreed to take the case and that the retaining agreements are in place. The usual next step begins with your receipt of written materials on the case, often in orange crate–sized lots. In other cases, your first task might be an evaluation of plaintiff, defendant, testator, or even witness. Which comes first boils down to a matter of individual preference. Some experts favor the unbiased (and perhaps uninformed) first look at the examinee after having read only the complaint, followed by review of the documentation; others prefer to review records first as a means of shaping their interview focus later (further discussion of this issue occurs later in this chapter). Scheduling considerations may determine the first task; it may be easier to clear 2 hours for an interview than 5 to review a chart. In any case, the next task is clear.

Is the Case Valid? The Threshold Question

The first question posed to the expert because of the very nature of your consultative role is, does the side retaining you have a valid case (or even a case valid in at least some aspects on which decisions about litigation or settlement could be made)?

Note that in an ideal world, attorneys would call you only for ironclad solid cases in which they have every confidence. In reality, the attorney may be employing you in a desperate attempt to clutch at some faint hope. There is nothing inherently wrong with this desperation, because the attorney is obligated by ethical concerns to exert every effort to represent a client zealously and vigorously, including by obtaining expert consultation. However, the emotional pressure of the attorney's desperation should not alter your objectivity.

Does the Attorney Have Merit?

Regrettably, you must ask the question, does the attorney have merit? As a rule, you should determine what kind of attorney you will be working with: is this someone to whom you wish to be linked, even in a consultative sense? In the initial telephone call, I recommend listening for indexes of venality, a tendency to assume you will give the "desired" opinion no matter what the material shows, or a tendency to want to withhold information. Two of the most powerful red flags that warn you to divest yourself of this relationship are lying and arguing.

The point is perhaps an obvious one, but one of the best indicators about the integrity of retaining attorneys is whether or not they lie to you. For example, I was once retained to perform an independent examination of a patient who was considered for involuntary commitment, in relation to which, of course, his dangerousness was the crucial issue. The attorney presented the case to me by telephone, stating that the patient's dangerousness flowed from his being charged with slashing tires, behavior that certainly did not seem all that threatening, compared with some behavior. On perusing the old record, however, I found an earlier evaluation by a friend and colleague who is nationally known for his expertise in assessing dangerousness; my colleague described this patient as probably the most dangerous person he had ever seen in his forensic career, based on the patient's history of significant violence.

Somewhat annoyed, I telephoned the attorney and demanded to know why he had withheld this history. The attorney's response was pathognomonic: "Why do you guys always have to go for the history? Why can't you just take the person as he stands there and assess him as he is right then?" I elected to turn the case down. You cannot afford to embark on a course of work with someone such as this particular attorney. If he or she withholds or distorts information or lies to you initially, then you have to expect the same in the future; therefore, the only safe course is not to work with that attorney. Expert witness work is hard enough without bad faith. (Note also in this example the value of the previous record, a document often difficult to unearth but essential to the full evaluation.)

The second red-flag situation occurs when, after you have given your verbal report, based on your review of the database, you give your conclusions, which happen to be unfavorable to the retaining attorney's case. Most ethical attorneys, faced with this disappointing fact, will acknowledge that they agree or felt the same as you did but needed to use expert input to satisfy their own mandates or those of the client or the insurer. Another less knowledge-able group of attorneys will be educated by your discussion.

Some attorneys, however, will argue with you at this point, and the arguments fall into two categories. In the first, the *benign* category, the attorney wants to be sure you understand the import of certain data, wants to be certain you took note of a particular record entry or deposition statement, or wants to call your attention to some information that has not been included in the original materials (such as a private investigator's report that the attorney does not want to send you to preserve its privilege). In the second, the *malignant* category, arguments are the attorney's attempt to browbeat you into changing your mind. Obviously, such pressure should be resisted, and the result may be your withdrawal from the case.

Underlying this issue is a more fundamental challenge for the expert: how far to go in negotiating with the attorney as to the limits of your opinion. A delicate balance must be struck between reasonable flexibility about, for instance, the wording in which your opinion is couched and the substantive alteration of your opinion. For example, in a competence assessment of an elderly person, I told the attorney that she possessed "islands of competence." He wondered if that could be equally well expressed by "areas of competence." After mulling this over, I decided those were near enough equivalents, but I emphasized that he and I needed to be clear about the relative small size of those areas. Agreement was struck.

In another case, I had prepared a 22-page single-spaced report. Although delighted with this level of detail, the attorney had planned to give the report to the jury at one point and feared it would put them to sleep. The attorney asked for major cuts or deletions. I accepted this—one can always say less—as long as the attorney understood that I would still stand by, and testify to if asked, the remainder of the opinion. This suggestion was acceptable.

It is important to ask for everything from the attorney, even if some material is irrelevant and other parts are inadmissible. Your request should be global, regardless of what may be precluded by rules of evidence and discovery. One attorney nearly drove me mad by releasing dribs and drabs of material, under the specious rationale that this method would permit seeing the evolution of my opinion.

The "I've Got Nothing" Problem

Although you prefer to work on a case in which your opinion is robustly supported by the database, a situation sometimes occurs that requires special mention. This ethical dilemma occurs when the attorney says, for example, "Look, I think this guy is probably not insane, but I'd like you to do this evaluation on him anyway because I've got nothing. He was photographed doing the crime." It is perfectly appropriate for the *attorney* (who is obligated zealously to defend the client) to request your aid as long as he or she levels with you about the facts, but you have to make your own ethical decision about the circumstances under which you as a forensic expert should take on a case in such an "I've got nothing" scenario. Either undertaking or turning down such a case is a defensible position; it is up to you. However, you should consider some important points.

First, a critical question is whether the fact that the attorney admits to having nothing will mobilize inappropriate sympathy on your part and bias you in terms of trying to find something—*anything*—in the case, even data of dubious validity. This problem is a variant of a countertransference issue, if you will, directed not toward the patient or examinee but toward the attorney.

Second, after your report, you would expect the attorney to accept the limited contribution you may make (if indeed it is limited) and not to attempt to persuade you to amplify or distort your conclusions. Referral to another or an additional expert also may be indicated.

Reviewing Cases Critically

When the attorney sends you a crate of records and you review them, check the documents you receive against the cover letter to be sure you have everything you should. As you go through the documents, develop a list of documents that need to be supplied and devise a way to check these off once you have received them. I have found that attorneys for some reason often fail to send the exhibits to depositions; long pages of deposition testimony drone on about the exhibit, but you can only imagine it because the actual document has not been provided.

In general, I find it helpful first to read the complaint so that you know what the basic issues are. As you read the complaint, look critically for claims, facts, and connections that can be checked against the primary record data and flag those in some way; you are creating a checklist, each element of which may be confirmed or disconfirmed by other material in the database. Recall that a plaintiff can claim anything at first.

Second, I read the medical records and clinical material or the equivalent; third, the depositions or witness reports. The logic of this procedure in terms of shaping your thinking is to start with what is being complained of (civil) or questioned (for example, insanity in a criminal context), then to check the record to determine whether the complaint or issue has any validity, and next to check the depositions (to observe how people retrospectively reported the facts and explained their rationale) or other documents (such as witness reports to review what others observed). At this point, you also may want to review relevant literature on the subject, including your own.

I *strongly* recommend reading large chunks of material at a single sitting, no matter how difficult the scheduling might be. This approach is the best way to have the whole case in memory so that you can catch contradictions between different sections of the database.

Given the complexity of many psychiatric malpractice cases, you may find it worthwhile and cost-effective to create time lines for various events occurring during the same period. This permits, for example, matching medication changes to symptom reduction or an increase in social withdrawal to assessed suicide risk. A laptop computer for this task may be quite helpful.

The Interview

After reading the materials, if you have not already done so, you will want to interview the plaintiff, the defendant, the testator, the witness, or whoever is involved in the case (presumably, you are familiar with basic interview approaches). Note for completeness that some experts like to start by examining the litigant first, cold, or with only the complaint reviewed. Doing so provides a potentially valuable tabula rasa on which examinees may write what they will; your interview queries would thus arise directly out of the material. Such an examinee-first approach, however, makes it harder to focus on hot spots of the case or areas of contradiction in the database.

Some discretion, advance screening, and selection of a safe environment may be required for examining potentially dangerous examinees. It is probably wisest to allocate several hours for an initial examination and smaller blocks of time for later follow-up. The attorneys on the case may limit the interview time available; exert every effort through your attorney to obtain enough time to do an adequate examination. If the appropriate amount of time for your examination cannot be obtained, accept it as a limitation, and be prepared to acknowledge this constraint as a limitation on the data.

If the witness lives locally, it might be effective and appropriate to examine him or her first, then to read the database, then to examine him or her again to clear up matters raised by the written material. Examinees who must travel to see you should, as a rule, be spared this burden.

Note that when you are retained by the defense and wish to examine the plaintiff, that side's attorney may refuse to allow you to do so. This decision is legitimate but bears consequences; the absence of this datum must be factored into the opinion. For example, in one case, the plaintiff's attorney on cross-examination asked whether it was not true that my opinion was reached without my examining the plaintiff. My immediate response, "You wouldn't let me!," was appropriately disconcerting.

Not uncommonly, when examining for the opposite side of a

case, the expert will receive a request to have an attorney or para-legal present during the interview or, alternatively, to have the interview audiotaped or videotaped. Jurisdictional rules may make one or all of these procedures mandatory, but I strongly recommend opposing their occurrence through your attorney. The fundamental reasons are as follows:

1. These procedures distract you from being able to give full empathic attention and close observation to the examinee and, for some experts, inhibit free-ranging inquiry.
2. Inappropriate interruptions and objections, cuing, and suggestions from the attorney present may contaminate the process.
3. Examinees commonly play up to the audience or recording device, exaggerating symptoms, focusing on making a recording, or consciously attempting not to contradict what they told the attorney earlier rather than evincing spontaneous (and thus, presumably, more authentic) responses to your inquiries.

Under rare circumstances, an audiotape or videotape of an interview may be constructive; it is certainly beneficial for teaching and for self-review for quality assurance. Verbatim material also can be obtained in this way. However, unobtrusive note taking probably represents the optimum compromise among choices. Experts whose handwriting is truly hieroglyphic report some success with taking notes on laptops, although this irritates some examinees more than writing during the interview.

If you are unable to prevent the above intrusions, attempt to put recording devices out of direct sight (although you should obtain on the tapes themselves verbal permission to record) and attempt to have the attorney or paralegal sit silently out of vision (for example, behind the examinee). If the attorney attempts in any way to cue or coach the examinee, warn once; a second offense should lead you to terminate the interview and report this interference to your retaining attorney.

To offer a structure for this stage of the inquiry, the format that

I devised for assessing true or false allegations of sexual misconduct may be helpful here. The following are four of the principles that I apply as a generic framework for this purpose.

Plausibility.   The first question to ask of the case, be it civil or criminal, is whether the case is fundamentally plausible. Do the deviations from standard of care sound hokey, as when the complaint boils down to, "I could tell by the expression on my doctor's face that he was having sexual thoughts about me, and I want to sue him" or when a defendant with no history of mental illness whatsoever is advancing a case for legal insanity based on, "I wasn't myself when I plotted that elaborate armed robbery"?

Internal consistency.   Does the subject on the side retaining you present a coherent story, the parts of which do not refute one another? Did the subject tell the same story to different observers at different times or a varied story? What benign factors might account for this discrepancy? What might this finding imply about possible fabrication, distortion, and so on?

"Alibi" issues or external consistency.   Is there material from somewhere else that challenges or refutes the claim? Does the defendant claim to have been totally psychotic and out of control, whereas the arresting officers and other disinterested witnesses describe a calm and rational person just after the crime? Do other parts of the total database present corroboration or discorroboration of the claims, observations, or statements of others? Was either the plaintiff or the defendant out of town on a reasonable alibi at a critical point when negligence was claimed?

Alternative scenario.   The notion of the alternative scenario can be essential for civil claims, such as sexual misconduct, or for some criminal claims, as well as disability evaluations and similar tasks. If the situation did *not* occur in the manner claimed, how might it have occurred alternatively? Is there another way of explaining what happened, the outcome, or the alleged damages? For example, is the disability due to an actual mental disorder or an avoidance of work for defensive reasons? Is the examinee attempting some sort of retaliation against the defendant for some perceived offense or slight other than that which is claimed?

Given the perpetual problem of malingering and baseless claims that are part of the backdrop of every forensic assessment, all of the foregoing questions can be kept in mind to aid in probing each case as you examine the database.

Finally, remember not to offer any treatment or treatment recommendations to your examinee, even if asked to do so or tempted by medical necessity as treatment issues emerge in the interview. The relationship is not a medical one, and treatment offers are inappropriate.

Fitting Together the Interview

Commonly, in both civil and criminal cases, you will interview the subject (plaintiff, defendant, and others) as part of your exhaustive review of the database. You will be challenged to weave interview data into the totality of the case, and you must keep several issues in mind.

First—you can't be reminded of this too often—is warning the examinee about nonconfidentiality. Other warnings, such as informing the examinee which side has retained you, seem to be called for out of fundamental fairness to your examinee. The following is an example of warnings that I (you may want to craft your own) give to examinees just after "hello, please sit down" but before anything substantive has been said:

> Before we start, there are some things I need to inform you about. First, unlike what you may be familiar with from other doctors or therapists, what we talk about here is not confidential because I am not your treater; what you say may come out in a report, in a deposition, or in an open courtroom. Second, I have been retained by (your side or the other side of the case), but since I can only be useful if I am objective, my testimony may help your case, hurt your case, or have no visible effect on your case—only time will tell. Third, you can ask for a break (water, rest room) at any time. And fi-

nally, you do not have to answer any of my questions, although I hope you will do so. Do you have any questions about what I have told you so far?

If the person has questions, answer them as best you can; if not, move on to the substance of your interview. Note the fully intentional structural resemblance of the above paragraph to informed consent.

As you are interviewing the examinee, you are attending to his or her demeanor and its relation to credibility. Is the patient convincing and plausible? Do the words match the music; that is, does the content resonate with the affect or is there discontinuity? Does the story told in the interview match the remainder of the database?

For perspective, recall that anyone can really be fooled. I remember a particular case of alleged sexual misconduct in which the plaintiff on interview absolutely convinced me with every single word she said. Her emotions were strong and appropriate to the content; she had plausible answers for all my questions. Only when I subsequently read her deposition did her entire case fall apart. Besides serving as a valuable lesson in humility, the case was highly instructive: interviewees can be extremely convincing, especially when they themselves, because of their psychopathology, believe deeply in their position. Remember the ancient received wisdom: if you are dealing with a classic psychopath and you think you are not being conned, it only means that you're being conned into thinking that you're not being conned.

The Causation or Connection Dilemma

In many forensic cases, the presence of a mental illness per se or the presence of emotional injuries is not particularly in doubt. What is more uncertain is the link—causation or connection—between those clinical details and the forensic issue. For example, a defendant may be mentally ill, but did that illness meet the statutory criteria for insanity? The treater may have deviated from the standard of care, but did that deviation cause the damages, or were other factors involved?

Examine previous or preexisting illness or injury to obtain valuable background. An insanity claim may be far more plausible when the patient has a long history of bona fide mental illness, but recall that anyone may have a "first psychotic break" with symptoms that meet insanity criteria. A claim for injury by an event in the recent past is more convincing when no preexisting emotional disorders are involved. This issue is further discussed in Chapter 4 in this volume.

The evaluating expert must resolve a delicate tension in determinations regarding previous or preexisting conditions. This is the question of whether previous symptomatology constitutes the plaintiff's "thin skull" (that is, particular plaintiff vulnerability for which the defendant must be held responsible, in the context of the basic legal concept in tort law of "taking the plaintiff where you find him or her") or whether, on the other hand, the preexisting condition must be deducted from the damages, because the defendant is not causally responsible for what happened earlier. An intermediate dilemma is that in which the defendant's alleged actions exacerbated (but did not originally cause) the preexisting harm. Such distinctions are extremely significant in the hard monetary realities of the legal case.

Similarly problematic is the matter of intervening causes: "Dr. Smith did X at this point, but then Dr. Jones did Y." In the civil system, plaintiffs are supposed to take steps to mitigate (ameliorate or diminish) their harms, but those efforts may fail or be misdirected and may even make things worse.

One of the most challenging tasks for the expert is to peel apart the sequence of events to determine what the results were of a particular deviation, event, or incident; what the results were of subsequent events; and what the exacerbations were of preexisting conditions. A familiar example is the case in which a plaintiff has been the survivor of severe sexual abuse in childhood with consequent symptoms, then is sexually abused by a treater, and then has other symptoms or more of the same symptoms. Or, consider a veteran of combat with posttraumatic stress disorder from wartime experience who is injured in an automobile accident sometime later. What portion (usually, what amount and what percentage) of the damages can be assigned to the later trauma?

To take this issue out of the guessing-game arena, work by Pittman and Orr (2) shows promise, although it has not yet gained broad enough acceptance to be generally admissible as evidence. These authors have devised a psychophysiological test protocol that offers some hope of distinguishing among traumas. Further research may reveal other promising approaches (3).

Keeping Records

How long should you keep records? A basic rule is that you should never discard case materials until you have asked the retaining attorney if you can do so. Even if a case seems "over," there may be subsequent posttrial motions, appeals, mistrial claims, and so forth that require revisiting the materials.

Another good rule is to discard, with permission, all case materials except your reports, if any, and your interview notes; keep the latter indefinitely, because they would be hard to replace. In addition, they may serve you to recall the case at a later point for research or publication purposes.

References

1. Kirby v Ahmad, 63 Ohio Misc 2d 533 at 534, 1994
2. Pittman RK, Orr SO: Psychophysiologic testing for post-traumatic stress disorder: forensic psychiatric application. Bull Am Acad Psychiatry Law 21:37–52, 1993
3. Bursztajn HJ, Feinbloom RI, Hamm RM, et al: Medical Choices, Medical Chances: How Patients, Families and Physicians Can Cope With Uncertainty. New York, Routledge, Chapman, Hall, 1990

Suggested Readings

Bloom JD, Bloom JL: The consultation model and forensic psychiatric practice. Bull Am Acad Psychiatry Law 13:159–164, 1985

Borum R, Otto R, Golding S: Improving clinical judgment and decision-making in forensic evaluation. Journal of Psychiatry and Law (Spring): 33–76, 1993

Group for the Advancement of Psychiatry, Committee on Psychiatry and Law: Report 131: The Mental Health Professional and the Legal System. New York, Brunner/Mazel, 1991

Lees-Haley PR: Attorneys influence expert evidence in forensic psychological and neuropsychological cases. Assessment (in press)

Lees-Haley PR, Williams CW: Response bias in plaintiffs' histories. Brain Inj (in press)

4

Types of
Typical Cases

To illustrate some of the principles highlighted in preceding chapters, in this chapter, I provide some examples of cases—and some of the nuances unique to each type of case—that clarify the spectrum of the expert's work. The discussions within this chapter should be considered an introductory survey.

Psychiatric Malpractice Cases

One of the most critical issues in psychiatric malpractice is the failure to prove all four elements of malpractice (dereliction of a duty directly causing damages). But the jury must face an even more challenging task in hearing the case long after the events occurred: the hindsight bias. Generally, the hindsight bias refers to the fact that everybody's retrospective view is 20/20. More practically, this bias means that the outcome of events appears as though it had been far more foreseeable, once you know it has already happened, than was actually so before the event in question occurred.

In a suicide malpractice case, for example (the most common claim against mental health professionals), you already know the person is dead; every potential signal of suicide becomes charged with inappropriate significance because the outcome is known. Sometimes forgotten is the foresight perspective, namely, that literally thousands of patients express suicidal ideas or hints *without* acting on them and that the suicide base rate is low. Like juries, you—even as an expert—can be vulnerable to the same hindsight-driven distortion of reasoning unless you actively work on countering this potential bias, usually by attempting empathically and effortfully to place yourself in the mind-set of the decision makers at past points in time when critical interventions did or did not occur. It takes active work and a creative imagination to get yourself into the *prospective* view of the foresight-driven treater, whose behavior must be measured against the standard of care as if the outcome were still in doubt (which, at an earlier time, it usually was). The task for the defense expert, and the ethical position for the plaintiff's expert, requires explaining to the jury exactly that retrospective yet foresight-oriented view (1–3).

A concept closely related to the avoidance of hindsight bias is that of respect for the primacy of the on-site observer. In psychiatric malpractice cases, it is most fair to the defendant (whichever side you represent) to weight heavily the fact that the defendant-physician, not yourself, was on the scene at the relevant time and under the applicable circumstances. This uniqueness of locale has a number of implications, all of which militate in favor of the on-site observer being given the benefit of the doubt in most observations and decisions, absent gross deviations from the standards of care.

One basis for this perspective is the matter of subjective data (4, 5). In addition to what is recorded in the chart, the direct observer who talked to this patient before he or she committed suicide had access to far more information than usually makes it onto the chart page: tone of voice, body language, facial expression, observer signs (the psychophysiological responses the patient evokes in the examiner), and similar subjective but often decisive elements of the decision-making process in regard to this patient. You, in contrast, have only the secondary materials (such as charts and depositions). Note that attorneys' queries in depositions about the aforementioned subjective observations are practically unheard of.

Although there is some variation annually, the leading issues in malpractice claims against psychiatrists over the years have been the following: suicide, sexual misconduct and boundary issues, third-party claims (that is, *Tarasoff*-type cases), confidentiality breaches, medication issues, and "false memory" cases in various forms. Many of these are subsumed within other categories such as misdiagnosis, mistreatment, wrongful death, and the like.

With the foregoing in mind, we can appreciate that it is a mark of the novice (or, alas, the venal) expert to say, "I have read the record, and *I know* the patient was depressed," despite the fact that the on-site observer records a careful mental status examination *without* reference to depression. Of course, it is quite a different matter if the on-site treater's conclusions are internally inconsistent with his or her own contemporaneous observations or are egregious distortions of the diagnostic or therapeutic process. But absent such extremes, great primacy should be awarded to subjective, nondocumented material that is observed by the on-site personnel at the relevant time.

It is therefore important to suspend your judgment while reading a case until the whole has been reviewed. Each side can be surprisingly convincing when assessed in a vacuum (such as the complaint or interview alone) so that premature closure of your opinion is a great hazard of the trade. Resist this temptation, and flag those claims that need to be checked against other parts of the database.

The Standard of Care

The question of the standard of care is a complex but central issue in malpractice; it is the benchmark against which deviation (that is, negligence) is measured. Unfortunately, the official standard of care or the wording in which it is couched may vary between jurisdictions. As an expert, you must of course familiarize yourself with the relevant local standard and its wording early in your work on the case and apply it to your review of the database. Massachusetts case law, for example, has a rather elaborate definition; the standard of care is that of "the average reasonable practitioner at that time and under the circumstances and taking into account the advances in the field." By inference, this is a national standard, because advances in the field are professionwide, not regional.

Other jurisdictions may have what is called a locality rule, which is a standard drawn from the practice of clinicians in that locality. For example, part of my qualification process in testifying in Durham, North Carolina, which has the locality rule, was to demonstrate the various ways in which I was aware of what clinicians do in Durham.

In light of some recent American Psychiatric Association (APA) publications articulating diagnostic and treatment guidelines, how are these guidelines to be construed in relation to standards of care? The average guideline is not itself a standard; rather than describing average actual practice, the guideline often identifies what care ideally should be. For example, if you write a textbook of psychiatry and law that proposes certain recommendations, those are not the standard of care. Those recommendations are called precatory or preaching; that is, they preach what the best care should be. Those recommendations do not pretend to be the standard of the average reasonable practitioner. All of these citations are legally considered "evidence of the standard," which the judge or jury may consider with other evidence.

In practice, you will be trying to find your way among these alternative models—none of which is the standard of care. Be prepared to answer the critical question, "Doctor, how do *you know* what is the standard of care?" and be prepared to be challenged on this point. Some common sources for obtaining this knowledge include conversations with colleagues, national professional meetings such as the APA annual meeting, national professional journals, and even previous forensic cases that have been tried in the same state or region or those that have involved comparable clinical issues.

Some subtleties remain. The expert may practice in an academic center at the cutting edge of research and practice, causing a potential biasing factor. Is the standard of care different for a resident and a senior practitioner? Probably. Is it different for a major urban academic teaching hospital and a small rural nonteaching one? Probably. How, then, can a fair and responsible accommodation to this difference be made? How do you assess it? Whatever your answer, do it fairly and be prepared to defend the rationale.

Further Notes on Reading the Records in Malpractice Cases

Records are frequently the core of the case. It is important not only for malpractice defense but also for rendering clinical care that the records are readable, logical, clinical, and internally consistent. The expert should, of course, screen for these qualities in reviewing them.

But the forensic level of scrutiny requires deeper probing. For example, is there symmetry between the clinician's notes and his or her orders, and the clinician's notes and the nurses' notes, the laboratory slips, the tests ordered, and so on? Are the appropriate countersignatures present if needed? Such comparative reading often distinguishes expert review in malpractice from utilization or peer review, for example.

An important principle in reading records cannot be reemphasized too often: never read a record (or for that matter, any forensic document) without making some sort of notation of what is significant, of your thoughts and reactions, of any queries that the record generates to be checked later or elsewhere, of what this record entry contradicts or supports in the deposition, or whatever. This notation can be on a separate sheet of paper of similar notes, or it can be a highlighted entry, a marginal scribble, an underline, a folded corner of the page, or a similar notation. In the process of reading, you may be tempted to say to yourself, "This is so clear and memorable that I will naturally recall it later." However, the next time you read this document for deposition or trial may be 7 *years* away. To save yourself reading everything from scratch each time, make some sort of notation each time you read through the record, as different things may strike you on subsequent review.

Because keeping a medical record is itself part of the standard of care, the expert may draw conclusions from the record alone, even in the face of other testimony by treaters or similar persons that extends or contradicts what is written. It is not uncommon for some discrepancy to exist between the written record and later testimony—a discrepancy that the expert should weigh.

I find it valuable to look at the social service history, if present, as a separate document. I have been impressed by how often the social service history supplies additional relevant data or gives a more detailed and comprehensive family history than does the psychiatric history. It is useful to compare the perceptions of the social worker (who often has worked extensively with the family) with the perceptions of other staff.

Next, after the records, you read the depositions of witnesses, plaintiffs, defendants, opposing experts, and others. The intrinsic problem is that the deposition usually takes place long after the incident occurred and certainly after litigation has been initiated (a problem that potentially biases or distorts the issues, of course). When reading the deposition, you are seeking consistency and credibility, as well as reasonable rationales or arguments that can be presented and explained at a greater length than possible in most patient charts.

The point may seem obvious, but depositions consist of *attorneys'* questions to various parties; these may not necessarily be the questions you would want to ask, nor are the queries necessarily posed the way you would do so. There is something of a translation burden on you to read between the lines to determine the issues. On some occasions, you may have to pose your own questions directly to the parties, through your retaining lawyer's permission and intercession.

Although the more information gathered, the more helpful it

would be in forming your opinion, it is inappropriate to call or write directly to the opposing attorney, litigant, or expert. All communications beyond the most mechanistic (giving the opposing attorney's secretary directions to your office for a deposition) should be channeled through your attorney.

On occasion, I have had opposing attorneys telephone me directly to see what they could get me to disclose about a case without the trouble and expense of scheduling a deposition. These unethical conversations usually have an informal tone: "So, Doctor, what do you think about this amazing case, eh?" Presumably, you are lulled by this informal, friendly approach into letting your guard down and discoursing freely on your opinions, your attorney's confidential trial strategy, and so on. The appropriate response is, "I think you should talk to the retaining attorney." Attorneys who push this issue should be reported to their local bar association's ethics committee.

Because of the flow of material and its often fascinating content, while reading a deposition, you can be drawn into the prose by the unfolding drama therein recorded. To read critically, exert the effort to stand back from the record, weighing the logic of the deponent's responses.

Criminal Responsibility Cases

In cases of criminal responsibility, you may confront the classical poles of the issue, namely, a case wherein the defendant had or has a major, credible mental illness (and therefore a likely defense) versus a case with none of these qualities for which application of the insanity defense represents a desperate attempt by the attorney because all other defenses are precluded. The truly challenging case lies between these extremes. For example, you may have a palpably mentally ill individual whose illness still does not meet the statutory criteria, or you may have an apparently mentally healthy individual whose subtle disorder impinges precisely on the requisite capacities. In those jurisdictions where the issue exists, remember to consider diminished capacity as an intermediate condition.

Out of the entire panoply of available material on a criminal responsibility case, data gathered at the time of the alleged act, in my (and almost everyone's) view, are the most significant. These would include witness and victim reports, statements of the arresting officers, and records of any treating clinicians from points close in time to the alleged acts.

Of second-rank importance, but still relevant, is historical material, especially that which establishes the presence of persistent and relevant patterns of behavior or disorder. Is this defendant someone who seemed to show for the first time the presence of schizophrenia at age 54 just *after* he or she committed the bank robbery, or did he or she have a long history of mental illness with recurring hospitalizations and delusional symptoms that relate directly to the alleged act?

Finally, although mandatory and irreplaceable, the interview in a criminal responsibility case has the least power of all the data collected, largely because its after-the-fact timing and the inevitable self-serving elements of the defendant's position cloud the objectivity of the examination. The most valuable dimension of the interview is obtaining previously unrecorded history and the defendant's own self-reported rationale for his or her actions and own description of the internal mental state at the time of the act. All the interview data must be fitted to the totality of the database, as with all forensic evaluations.

Because of the seriousness of criminal penalties, malingering is especially common and problematic in this assessment. The novice expert should become familiar with useful publications on the subject (6, 7). Courses on detection of malingering are offered at national meetings of the APA and the American Academy of Psychiatry and the Law.

Evaluation of Emotional Injuries

In contrast to the interview for a criminal responsibility case, I find the interview for an emotional injury case to be of primary value.

Nothing but the interview can give you a feeling for the malingering dimension and the self-serving aspects of the patient's claim. The interview also gives you a chance to assess what might be called a sense of proportion. The plaintiff who claims that his or her major posttraumatic stress disorder (PTSD) and all of his or her subsequent emotional problems were caused by a tiny bottle of vodka falling out of an airplane's overhead compartment might raise some issues of proportion.

This issue of proportion is a common pitfall for the novice plaintiff's expert, who may be tempted out of sympathy for the injured examinee to extend damages excessively from a limited injury. In one case, for example, a plaintiff drank from a chemically contaminated bottle and burned his mouth, an injury from which he recovered rapidly without lasting effect. The plaintiff's expert opined that being burned by an ostensible cooling drink had shaken the plaintiff's faith in a benign universe.

Although plaintiffs have an obligation to mitigate (reduce or ameliorate) their damages, a surprising number of individuals avoid treatment, some on their own and some when given this advice by their attorneys. A question you should ask your interviewee is, "What would have to happen for you to go get treatment to mitigate your damage in this area?" A response such as "I would have to find a doctor I liked" is quite reasonable; however, an answer such as "What is the point? There is no hope for me!" is more problematic (perhaps flowing from a depression) and suggestive of a need for some intervention before the examinee undertakes mitigation.

Focus on emotional damages from a particular event or situation should not blind you to exploration of personality or character issues. Not only might these provide a context for the injuries claimed, but they may be relevant to assessing damages or preexisting conditions.

History, too, especially idiosyncratic history, may be relevant. For example, consider the so-called strip search case in which store employees suspect the plaintiff of shoplifting goods and perform an embarrassing or inappropriately confrontational public search or semi-strip search, only to find that the goods are legitimately accompanied by a receipt. The shopper then may sue the store for harassment and consequent emotional harms. Such a search can be embarrassing and humiliating to anyone, but you might discover on questioning the plaintiff that the extreme subsequent trauma and dysfunction flow from a history of sexual abuse or public exposure and humiliation. This history may represent the plaintiff's "thin skull" (that is, preexisting vulnerability). In this situation, you again often encounter the previously described problem of factoring out the effects of serial trauma.

Finally, the expert is obliged to attempt to factor out those stresses and resultant symptoms of the litigation process itself—a challenging but necessary task.

Some examples of personal injury cases in which I have been involved may provide instructive insights into the evaluation process. These brief commentaries on some familiar types of cases are intended to fill in areas of the evaluation that standard texts may not address.

The Startle Response That Wasn't

A plaintiff had experienced a documented mugging and was suing the company for inadequate security. He claimed to have full-fledged PTSD, with intrusive flashback memories, avoidance, and startle responses, as a result of the mugging. I had to interview him in his home because he claimed to be phobically homebound. The interview took place in his basement recreation room. Next to the small table where we were sitting, there was a slatted wall or room divider that evidently concealed his home's heating apparatus. I knew this because, without warning, the heat abruptly went on with a loud "WHOOOMPP!" making a considerable racket right next to our chairs. I myself jumped in my chair, but I couldn't help noticing that my alleged startle examinee sat quietly in his chair.

This observation was potentially valuable and worth recording. It is of course not totally probative because he clearly might have been more accustomed and therefore conditioned to the noise of the heat going on, yet the observation is valid; the jury ultimately decides.

The Case of Cockroach Harm

Can infestation by cockroaches be a trauma? At low levels, usually not, but at incredibly high levels, perhaps so. One of my cases raised this issue. An apartment dweller sued her landlord for failing to respond to the infestation. A powerful factor in the assessment was a series of photos of the hordes of dead vermin lying about after the apartment in question had been gassed—a picture that was highly convincing.

The Story of the Stoic Fisherman

This case addresses the question of whether all traumas are traumatic. In a famous incident, an airplane skidded on an icy runway and broke in half at Boston's Logan Airport; the nose of the plane fell into the harbor. A passenger from that plane came to me for an examination in relation to a lawsuit for emotional injuries against the airline.

This passenger, it turned out, had been in the front row of seats just behind the break in the plane. He was strapped into his seat, and looking straight down past his toes, he saw a jagged metal edge and below that edge, Boston Harbor. On the surface of his story, it seemed to me that this incident would induce PTSD in a stone statue; therefore, the case certainly seemed meritorious in theory.

On examination, however, the former passenger was revealed as a serious, unimaginative, stoic fisherman, who, on careful inquiry, had *no* signs of trauma whatsoever. He slept like a log, ate like a lumberjack, and did not dream. He gave the impression on interview that if you fired off a .357 Magnum close to his ear, he would have said calmly, "What was that noise?"

This case illustrates the maxim, don't assume—examine, to get the actual data.

High-Profile Cases

At one point or another, you may be asked to review a case that has been extensively covered in the media before you have been retained; that is, the alleged malpractice, injury, or crime has generated publicity first, then you get the case. There is a fundamental asymmetry about media coverage in almost every case, which the average member of the public really doesn't understand: initially, the plaintiff or prosecutor can say anything. As the "moving parties," the attorneys have to create the case from scratch; there is no case until it is brought. Some attorneys may try, consciously or unconsciously, to influence the public powerfully in advance, in hopes that some of that public will later become jurors.

A plaintiff can say to the media, for example, "McDonald's has a duty to weld on the covers of coffee cups with Krazy Glue so that people can't hold them in their laps, rip them off in moving cars, and spill hot coffee over their thighs and sue McDonald's." In another case, a prosecutor may state to the media that the defendant's 23-year state hospitalization for schizophrenia was probably malingering and certainly has no bearing whatsoever on the insanity issue. None of this trumpeting means anything, of course, until it is proven in a court of law, but this principle may be readily overlooked in a media frenzy.

In short, plaintiffs and prosecuting attorneys can create any possible scenario they think they can prove. Ninety-nine percent of the time, however, the defense attorneys cannot answer the media's questions. The defense attorneys must say "no comment" each time because they don't want to give away trial strategy. This response creates asymmetry whereby the plaintiff and prosecutor totally dominate the media, pushing the case for all it is worth. By doing this, the plaintiff and prosecutor inevitably bias the public's perception.

Even though you may try to tune out the media, you simply may be reading your newspaper before you are asked to consult on a case. Therefore, you have to be alert to this potential biasing factor and be aware of the media asymmetries, lest your review should begin with a one-sided perspective.

Spotting the Other Side's "Hired Gun"

The hired gun problem is a cross borne by the forensic professions, as is outlined in Chapter 1 in this book. Recognizing this blot on our collective escutcheon will prepare you to deal with or counter the actions of the hired gun in court or elsewhere.

Does advertising your services in *Lawyers' Weekly* automatically make you a hired gun? This controversial question skirts perilously close to a matter of guilt by association. Probably a certain number of totally ethical people do advertise in *Lawyers' Weekly* but so do a number—perhaps a greater number—of venal witnesses, selling testimony instead of time. (Chapter 9 in this volume provides more reliable methods of publicizing your practice.)

Another stigma of the hired gun is the counsel of perfection. In malpractice cases, for example, the standard references the *average* reasonable practitioner—not the stars of the profession or those at the bottom of the barrel but those occupying the middle of the Gaussian curve. The hired gun often advances a perfectionistic standard as though it were the average. "If the care had been adequate, this suicide would not have occurred" is a proper statement of the relationship of causation to the standard of care, but "This suicide proves inherently that the care was inadequate" is a hindsight-driven standard of perfection. Such statements may even mask the fact that the hired gun does not know what the standard of care actually is.

Another variation on this theme is, "They (the defendants) should have done more." This testimony is a classic hired gun claim. Anyone always *could have* done more, but no one lives real life like that. The real issue is does the standard of care *require* more. Indeed, the counter to such claims often begins with the phrase "Well, in the real world. . . . " Many "good ideas" theoretically might have contributed to the patient's care, but malpractice litigation hinges on what is *required* by the standard of care.

Yet another variant on this last theme is the situation in which the hired gun advances his or her own idiosyncratic standard as the standard of care: "I always do X on every examinee I've ever seen." Note that what any particular expert does is irrelevant to determining the standard of care of the average reasonable practitioner.

Some experts believe that physicians are never wrong and always justify whatever the physicians do. Novice experts must avoid this possible pitfall by remaining alert to an overidentification with the treating physicians.

An even more malignant twist is the made-up or artificial standard. The hired gun whips a standard out of thin air to justify his or her position in the case. For example, one treater-cum-expert in a North Carolina case claimed that the standard of care required a psychiatrist who precipitously terminated treatment with a stalker (but made an appropriate referral and transfer) to embark—despite her personal fears—on a series of termination meetings with the stalker. I personally have never heard of or read that standard anywhere; the likely explanation is that the treater-expert made it up to suit his views of this case.

Another phenomenon you might see in the deposition that captures the notion of the hired gun is the "major waffle." The following is a real-life sample:

> *Examining attorney:* Does the standard of care require restraint of this patient?
> *Hired gun witness:* When you have a patient who is this out of control and depressed, it's a very serious situation, and you have to respond and give the patient what he needs or otherwise you'll have a really bad situation.
> *Examining attorney:* But does the standard of care require that this patient be restrained?
> *Hired gun witness:* I've already answered that.

That was the answer in toto. Is that a yes or a no? In fact it is neither—it is a waffle, and that is frequently the hallmark of the hired gun. Getting the feel for how the waffle works takes a certain amount of reading of case material.

Here is another example of a waffle on standard of care:

> *Question:* So you think after his discharge from [X Hospital] in [month] of [year], he should have been [that is, the standard of care required that he be] in-

voluntarily admitted to a hospital before [month] of
[year]?

Answer: It is my opinion that one of the possibilities
that should have been seriously considered would
have been an involuntary hospitalization. It certainly should have been considered. I am not in a
position to tell you that that would be the only
choice.

Note how that witness actually avoids responding; "should have
been seriously considered" is not an opinion that commitment in
this case was a *required action* under the standard of care. Also
note that the failure to consider a valid option indeed may constitute negligence, but that is the answer to a different question.

In the following example, a patient had escaped from the hospital, then committed suicide. The plaintiff's expert answers the
query as to the bases for his opinion that treatment was below the
standard of care. The entire answer took four full deposition
pages, but this excerpt is representative:

The standard of care in my professional opinion was breached in that
once the patient left, the mental state and what's gone on in that
patient's mind is very uncertain, that this is a patient with some history
of a, a reasonable history, actually, of unpredictability; he gets fright-
ened, he has taken in despair 10 lithiums some years back, took some
blood pressure pills one time in [city], goes all the way to [another
city], we don't know whether he stops or doesn't stop and get [drug]
or not, but, specifically, there is a lot of despair and a great deal of
thought disorganization in the patient, and where I believe the standard of care was breached was that the patient, an emergency petition
ideally would have been, reasonably would have been, rather than
ideally, reasonably should have been issued so that the patient could
be brought back for reassessment in terms of their thinking and what
possessed the patient to leave, an hour before that or less signs a 3-day
statement and then just disappears.

Note that this entire chunk of testimony is one run-on sentence;
parsing its grammar would be an excellent torture for an evil

grammarian consigned to hell. More to the point, it seems nearly impossible to extract the actual opinion from the thicket of prose.

The following is part of a response to a request to list deviations from the standard of care in a *Tarasoff*-type case:

> It's a consequential piece of behavior that creates the most essential elements of a treatment plan, which makes sure the patient is safe within a structured environment, and that includes they would be safe within or without the community, because the treatment will eventually take place if it can at all within a less restrictive alternative that is community based, but that doesn't mean that it's without supervision.

In fairness, we must consider another possibility regarding the above examples. I would prefer never to assume malice when incompetence would serve as an alternative scenario. Conceivably, we may be dealing with an incompetence issue, whereby the deponents simply do not know how to focus on a forensic question. Yet, for better or for worse, a trend of such waffling answers in deposition does set off my hired gun detector.

References

1. Gutheil TG, Bursztajn H, Brodsky A, et al: Decision-Making in Psychiatry and Law. Baltimore, MD, Williams & Wilkins, 1991
2. Fischhoff B: Hindsight, foresight: the effect of outcome knowledge on judgment under uncertainty. Journal of Experimental Psychology 1:288–299, 1975
3. Tversky A, Kahneman D: The framing of decisions and the psychology of choice. Science 211:453–458, 1981
4. Gutheil TG, Bursztajn H, Brodsky A: Subjective data and suicide assessment in the light of recent legal developments, I: malpractice prevention and the use of subjective data. Int J Law Psychiatry 6:317–329, 1983
5. Bursztajn H, Gutheil TG, Brodsky A: Subjective data and suicide assessment in the light of recent legal developments, II: clinical uses of legal standards in the interpretation of subjective data. Int J Law Psychiatry 6:331–350, 1983

6. Rogers R: Clinical Assessment of Malingering and Deception. New York, Guilford, 1988
7. Gothard S, Viglion DJ, Meloy JR, et al: Detection of malingering in competency to stand trial evaluations. Law and Human Behavior 19:493–505, 1995

Suggested Readings

Binder RL: Sexual harassment: issues for forensic psychiatrists. Bull Am Acad Psychiatry Law 20:409–418, 1992
Bolocofsky DN: Use and abuse of mental health experts in child custody determinations. Behavioral Sciences and the Law 7:197–213, 1989
Fitch WL, Petrella RC, Wallace J: Legal ethics and the use of mental health experts in criminal cases. Behavioral Sciences and the Law 5: 105–117, 1987
Scrigmar CB: Post Traumatic Stress Disorder: Diagnosis, Treatment and Legal Issues. New Orleans, LA, Bruno Press, 1988
Slovenko R: Legal aspects of post-traumatic stress disorder. Psychiatr Clin North Am 17:439–446, 1989
Stone AA: Post traumatic stress disorder and the law: clinical review of the new frontier. Bull Am Acad Psychiatry Law 21:23–36, 1993

5

Discovery and Depositions

During the extensive period between filing a suit or arresting
a suspect of a crime and the actual trial, if any, there is the period
known as discovery. Attorneys probe and define the limits of their
cases, preparing for what to expect from the various witnesses and
documents. Note that some jurisdictions practice "trial by ambush"
without expert discovery, whereby the other side learns for the
first time who is serving as the expert only when that individual is
called to the stand. Paralegals in those locales may call all major hotels the night before the trial to check on some likely names.

From the viewpoint of the expert, the two most common
mechanisms for the other side to discover projected expert testimony are interrogatories and depositions.

Interrogatories

Interrogatories as part of the discovery process are written responses under oath to a series of often standardized questions from the other side that may be used to elicit the names of witnesses and parties to a legal proceeding and an outline of what they might be expected to say. Under some circumstances, using interrogatories to inform the other side of the names of the expert witnesses is replaced by a letter or report called an expert disclosure. In both cases, the attorney will likely write the actual prose of the answers for you, the expert, guided by your input as to what you expect to testify to at trial.

Novice experts are sometimes tempted to regard this step as a mere formality and to pay it little heed, reasoning that they can always modify their opinions at trial when the right questions are asked. However, the interrogatory is sworn testimony, and an attorney may make a major issue out of any deviation in your trial testimony and what your interrogatory disclosure states that you will say.

The obvious prophylaxis and remedy is to attend carefully not only to the content of what your lawyer puts down as your expected testimony but also to the specific choice of words being used. It is critical that everything in your interrogatory be something that you have already decided you are able to support, either from clinical evidence or experience or from facts in the database. This approach saves you from having to retract misstatements on cross-examination. Resist any temptation to predict sweeping conclusions you might draw that go beyond your data; hyperbole hurts *you*.

In addition, your attorney will advise you as to what requests for information or documents will be objected to or refused, based on his or her interpretation of the rules of evidence. For example, attorneys sometimes ask you for your tax returns of the last 5 years, to which they are not entitled (although they are usually allowed to ask what percentage of your income comes from forensic work). Do not attempt to decide what is or is not objectionable yourself; that is an attorney's function.

Depositions

The second major area of discovery is the deposition. If you have never given a deposition or you feel a bit shaky about the procedure, review Chapter 5 in the companion volume to this book, *The Psychiatrist in Court: A Survival Guide.*

Opposing attorneys usually follow one of three agendas, or some combination of the three: getting your opinion, obtaining admissions, and painting you into a corner.

Getting your opinion.   First, there is the authentic wish to discover what your opinions at trial will be and what the bases for your opinions are, over and above what has been conveyed in reports or interrogatories, if any. The attorney can then prepare cross-examination, select rebuttal witnesses, inform his or her experts about facts or issues to pay attention to, and so on. This discovery function is a completely legitimate task and one with which you should cooperate fully.

Of course, the attorney is not averse to discovering precisely those points that will help his or her side of the case, but this is a subintention within the larger discovery framework.

Attorneys also stress that the deposition is their one chance to find out what you have to say. In this latter context, depositions are occasionally, but not ideally, taken before the entire database has been acquired or reviewed by the experts; time considerations, scheduling problems, and deadlines may dictate this suboptimal condition. When you subsequently receive, for instance, a witness's deposition or medical record that you had not seen before your own deposition, and—as a result of reviewing the facts or statements in that new document—your opinion materially changes in some way (other than merely being strengthened), you are ethically obligated to so inform your attorney, who is in turn obligated to inform the attorney on the other side of your new opinion. This information may or may not trigger a supplemental step for you in the form of an interrogatory, a telephone conference, or a full-fledged repeat deposition.

The obligation to give your opinions and bases for those

opinions in response to questions does not obligate you, however, to empty your word-hoard, as the Anglo-Saxons phrased it. Your crisp and focused answers do not require pouring out every thought you have ever had about the case, the attorney, the police, the plaintiff, the defendant, and so on. Just answer the question. On the other hand, attempts to ambush the other side at trial by testimony previously omitted may subject you to abuse on cross-examination for your duplicity in not giving that opinion during deposition.

Some cunning attorneys attempt to exploit this point by avoiding asking you relevant opinion questions at all. They try to restrict or even bar your testimony on the stand on the basis that you did not proffer those opinions on deposition. This ploy usually can be defused by your attorney, who may pose the key questions after the adverse attorney has completed his or her side of the deposition, as a way of ensuring that your opinions may be brought out at trial.

Obtaining admissions.   The second major agenda for the deposing attorney is to obtain from you, during the course of the deposition, admissions and concessions of points or views detrimental to the other (that is, *your*) side of the case. The points may relate to guilt, competence, insanity, negligence, or damages—the entire gamut of forensic possibilities. Indeed, many attorneys would view themselves as highly successful in this effort if they could only dilute the force of your opinion or obtain agreement with a point that is or even *sounds* close to a concession. Their rationale for this effort is that a jury may not be able to distinguish between *is* and *sounds like.* For example,

> A patient was committed because of threats, based on paranoid-sounding content, to kill co-workers. On arrival at the hospital, however, he denied to the admitting physician that he had any violent intent. His mental status was not particularly demonstrative of symptoms of mental illness, although the history, of course, raised many possibilities. In a wrongful commitment case against the hospital, the deposing attorney asked the hospital's defense expert whether the mental status indicated the presence of serious mental

illness. The answer was no. At trial, much was made of this testimony, even though it was the preadmission history, not the mental status by itself, that justified the admission.

Painting you into a corner.   The third common agenda for the deposing attorney is painting you into a corner, conceptually, so that your opinion is constrained or limited in a way that decreases its impact. This procedure elicits sworn testimony (that is, under oath). You are locked in to that testimony. When you later give testimony in court, also under oath, any contradiction is obviously damaging to your credibility: "You swore this now and that then; what *are* we to believe, Doctor?"

Your vigilance to being painted into a corner by the deposing attorney is justified by the fact that there are many subtle variations of this locked-in approach. The most familiar variations include attempting to get you to generalize about psychiatry and ignore the differences among the schools of thought within the field, attempting to get you to describe what *you* would do rather than focusing on what the standard of care requires, and attempting to get you to authenticate quotes from your published articles as though the present case were governed by those excerpts.

Your Goals for the Deposition

One scholar has described the witness's goals as truth, fairness, and accuracy (1). Truth, of course, is the final standard. Fairness indicates the need not to distort or exaggerate on either side of the issue but to maintain balance. Accuracy addresses the clarity of your vision in relation to the known facts in the case.

You should state that you want the written record of the deposition to do justice to your views, your opinions (and their limitations), and your planned testimony.

Some Practical Points

The need for concentration.   The concepts previously mentioned should make clear that a deposition is not a mere formality to be gotten out of the way and over with. Rather, it is an essential part of the evolution of a case and thus your role in it. To do your job, you must be rested, focused, alert, and vigilant at all times. Occasionally, an attorney will turn the deposition into an endurance contest to try to beat down your opinion by having fatigue erode your concentration. Prepare for this. Get enough sleep the night before the deposition, try to eliminate distractions, and insist on your freedom to take breaks as frequently as you need to maintain your attentive edge. If you do not go home after a deposition feeling tired and drained, you were probably not paying sufficiently close attention; intense concentration sustained over hours is hard work.

Listen to the question. Make sure the question you are answering is the one you were actually asked. If there is the slightest doubt, ask to hear it again or have it read back. If the question is compound or complex, ask that it be broken down.

On rare occasions, you can give a useful compound answer to a compound question, but it is risky. The following example illustrates that you may be playing with fire when offering compound answers:

> *Question:* Now, are you seriously telling this court that
> that sentence [quoted from an article] is one which
> instructs the forensic witness and the medical health
> treater that, in order to determine competence, they
> have to enter into a dialogue with their patient, that
> this is one of the ways in which you go about deter-
> mining competence? Is that your testimony?
> *Answer:* Well, let me answer all three components.
> First, yes, it is serious. I am serious. Second, the
> capacity to enter into a dialogue is considered by
> the Program in Psychiatry and the Law, which I co-
> direct, to be a way of determining competence in
> the clinical situation. And the third part of your
> question is, yes, this could be used to instruct
> both the forensic assessor and the treating clini-

cian as to a means of determining the capacity to
enter into informed consent.

Note, in the following example, the subtlety of the have-you-
stopped-beating-your-wife dimension of the dialogue. The case involved a sudden brutal murder of a staff member by a patient who
gave no advance indicators or warnings whatsoever.

> *Question (attorney for staff member):* . . . Knowing
> what we know today, can we agree that on [date of
> murder] you did not have a clear understanding of
> [patient's] propensity for violence? [Questioner as-
> sumes there was a propensity in the patient—a hind-
> sight view—hence, the case manager's lack of
> understanding might be negligent.]
>
> *Answer (by case manager):* I don't think I would agree
> with that, no. I don't—I wouldn't agree with you
> there.
>
> *Question:* So, it's your testimony that on [date] you
> did have a clear understanding of [patient's] pro-
> pensity for violence [and therefore are negligent
> because you did nothing about it]?

By imputing to the patient a hindsight-based propensity for
the violence only now known to have occurred, the questioning
attorney bypasses the critical issue of assessment and hangs the
witness on the horns of an unresolvable dilemma: you didn't
know, so you were negligent, or you knew and didn't act, so you
were negligent.

A more effective answer might have been, "The patient gave no
sign, warning, or evidence of a propensity for violence; therefore,
his act could neither be foreseen nor be prevented."

Note how the question is incorporated into the answer so that
the answer stands alone and is difficult to quote out of context.
Obviously, the witness should decline to answer yes or no to such
a question.

The following excerpt of testimony given by a naive fact witness, testifying 5 years after a suicide, reveals the hazards of too effusive and too extensive an answer to deposition questions.

> *Question:* Did you observe [patient] attending those meetings, or did you make that entry based on information given to you by others? [These are, of course, not the only possibilities.]
>
> *Answer:* Gee, I sure hope I saw him because I usually don't write things unless they are true. [This is not an answer to the question. It is unlikely, 5 years and hundreds of patients later, that the witness specifically remembers such a detail; the answer, "I don't recall," would be perfectly okay. In addition, making a chart entry based on what you were told by other staff —for example, from a previous shift—is universal practice. But this witness has set a standard for herself: "hope for truth."]
>
> *Question:* Is that the procedure in which you make notes; you write down what you have observed, not what others have told you? [The attorney tightens that very screw.]
>
> *Answer:* Right, right. Gee, any good nurse does that. [The witness sets her own standard of care, which might be used against her nursing colleagues. Her answer ignores the fact that the record does not always note the source of the clinical data.]

Yet another deposition tactic is what I call gerrymandering the data. The gerrymander was a mythical beast from a political cartoon about cutting up voting districts into tiny pieces to manipulate election patterns. Clinical data also can be cut into discrete segments to attempt to refute, challenge, or weaken certain conclusions (2).

For example, a patient with apparent bipolar disorder challenged an involuntary commitment. When seen, the patient manifested rapid press of speech, vulgarity, social obnoxiousness in various ways, paranoia, and grandiosity; moreover, a psychiatrist friend of the patient reported to the physician that she had long tried to get the patient treated for bipolar disorder. The deposing attorney inquired, "Does speaking fast mean you have bipolar disorder?" Each microsymptom was examined similarly to show that any one symptom, in a vacuum, did not constitute sufficient evidence of bipolar disorder (although, of course, the totality of symptoms did so).

Note that an excellent and self-contained answer to such a question or line of questions is, "In a vacuum, no." This answer responds directly to the question at hand but preserves the conclusion that the total gestalt made the diagnosis, not the individual element.

The pregnant pause. After the question is asked, pause a moment. Pausing allows you to replay the question in your head and to think about your answer. The pause also allows other attorneys to object, instruct you not to answer, insist on a time frame, and so on.

Also remember to listen carefully to the objection; your attorney may be trying to call your attention to something, or you might infer something useful from the type of objection posed. If your attorney says, "Objection, lack of time frame," reflect a moment on why the time frame might be important in relation to that particular question.

Answers. Deposition answers are drawn from a surprisingly shallow pool. They are, in essence, "yes," "no," "I don't know," "I don't recall," or a short narrative response that contains the question so that the response, in effect, cannot be quoted out of context. (See also Chapter 5 in the companion volume, *The Psychiatrist in Court: A Survival Guide.* Some key points made in that volume are the hazards of guessing, the trap of double negatives in the questions, incomprehensible questions, and the importance of speaking slowly, clearly, and carefully for the stenographer, whose written record will be the actual form of the deposition in all future contexts. If any of these summary phrases do not trigger recognition, review the corresponding discussions in the companion volume.)

Your answers must be verbal and aloud, because the stenographer cannot record winks, nods, shakes, shrugs, and other myoclonic responses.

Attorneys may sometimes interrupt your answer, usually accidentally, in the belief that your pause means you have finished, but sometimes they do so deliberately to distract you or to break your concentration. Do not tolerate this interruption. Insist on finishing your answer to your satisfaction.

If your concentration slips and you give an answer that you later believe was wrong or even misleading, immediately correct it on the record. To err is human, but leaving the error on the record means having to retract it on cross-examination.

Baker makes an excellent point about the precision of an answer in the following excerpt (1):

> The opposing lawyer may ask: "Doctor, have you [a radiologist] ever seen an X-ray fracture like this one?" The radiologist knows that every fracture is slightly different. Therefore, he could accurately answer in the negative. However, this would permit the opposing attorney to infer that the witness was not qualified to testify concerning this type of fracture. Therefore, the doctor might answer: "Well, in all my years of practice I have probably seen between 400 and 500 fractures similar to this one, but I can't say that any of them were [sic] precisely like this one, because no two fractures are exactly alike." (pp. F8–F9)

Certain locutions that are perfectly acceptable in casual conversation are either problematic or downright damaging in the deposition setting. An inexperienced expert inserted into the deposition testimony these parenthetical musings: "To be honest with you. . . . No, I tell a lie. . . . To tell the truth. . . . If I said that, I'd be lying." Of course, the entire deposition takes place under oath and under penalty of perjury. Therefore, these otherwise colorful colloquialisms must dismay the listener and raise questions about either the testimony or the seriousness with which it was delivered—both unfortunate concerns.

As a deponent witness, you are not supposed to consult with the retaining attorney in the middle of a pending question because this raises the specter of coaching. Two points about this problem should be kept in mind. First, if you are concerned specifically about a matter of privilege that may govern your answer, most jurisdictions will allow you to raise that issue for advice from your retaining attorney before you answer. Second, you may at any point consult with your own personal attorney if you have any questions whatsoever about an answer; the deposition may be paused for that consultation. When in doubt, exercise this option.

When to throw it away. In my consultative experience, I find that the most common error the beginning expert makes in a deposition is the failure to concede an obvious and irrefutable point out of misguided loyalty to his or her side of the case. In a suicide malpractice case, for example, where you are retained by the defense, the deposing attorney may ask, "Doctor, would you agree that a patient's suicidal ideation should be recorded in that patient's record?" The answer is yes. Quibbling over the possible exceptions or equivocating in some way helps no one. Remember that the failure to write something down may be below the standard of care, but the lack of the note did not cause the suicide. When the answer is that clear, make the concession; throw it away, and move on. It is not the defendant's negligence that is at stake in this situation but your credibility.

Blows after the bell. After a deposition has been going on for a while and you have maintained your concentration throughout, an attorney may look ostentatiously at his or her watch and say, "Just a few more questions, Doctor, and we'll be done." At that point, the novice witness relaxes and loses focus, thinking about dinner and work to do later. But the witness is also in danger of making concessions and giving poor answers to the subsequent slew of questions that the attorney, having inexplicably found his or her second wind, now begins to fire rapidly at the witness, still, of course, on the record. The moral here, in the colorful argot of the national pastime, is "It ain't over till it's over." Wait to relax only after the stenographer has put away the machinery.

Occasionally, an attorney may attempt to get some off-the-record insight literally in the doorway, not unlike some patients in psychotherapy whose doorway pauses—"oh, just one more thing"—contain vital material, but you know enough not to get involved in that "thing."

Curious questions. The absence of a jury and of a judge to rule on the appropriateness of questions sometimes gives deposing attorneys the feeling of freedom to ask questions that might be disallowed by a judge or be seen as impertinent by a jury. Questions of morality and values—areas that are outside of forensic psychiatric expertise—fall into this category: "Doctor, was the widow wrong to do what she did?" or "Was this defendant wrong to feel a desire for revenge?" or "Is that something a child might think?" (assuming you are not a child psychiatrist).

The only valid answer is that those questions are outside your area of expertise, and this response is perfectly appropriate. A surprising number of expert witnesses appear to have no qualms about tackling moral questions about which they have firmly fixed ideas; they often fail to realize that they do not have *forensic evidence* to back up those notions.

Some questions are curious because the attorney appears to be flailing at, rather than asking about, the subject matter. Responding to such flails is a challenge:

> *Question:* In that case [of suicide in an alcoholic man], using categorization, if you're grossly suicidal and you have access to guns and drugs and alcohol, isn't it a greater hazard to you as a person doing those things—and isn't it a fact your duty at that point as a psychiatrist arises [sic] to a higher level because of your knowledge of these conditions?
>
> *Answer:* You lost me. . . .
>
> *Question:* Isn't it true that sensitivity to the humanness of our problem is one that needs to be dealt with in a medical field, that we can't isolate ourselves with notions of "I'm not part of our society," in a manner to ignore those feelings, those underpinnings? Isn't

that sensitivity what separates a real doctor from a
phony doctor?

Answer: Well, I find your question a little confusing,
but I'm in favor of sensitivity.

Note how the first question was a total loss and had to be re-
jected completely. The answer to the second question illustrates a
sometimes useful technique: extract that fragment of usable answer from the chaos if you can, and answer that part. This method
sometimes involves carefully answering the question that the attorney *should* have asked; make sure you include the question in
your answer on those occasions so that no one is misled.

The limits of expertise.   Indeed, acknowledging the limits of
what you can say constitutes one of the ethical benchmarks for the
expert. No expert is expected to be an expert in everything or to remember everything; therefore, "I don't know" or "I don't remember" is a fully appropriate answer, as is "That is outside my area of
expertise." Avoid the narcissistic trap of "I can answer anything."

Deposition demeanor.   The ideal posture for the deponent expert is only slightly different from that on the witness stand: calm,
firm, clear, unfailingly polite, never losing your cool. The only vital
difference is the way in which you speak. Because the stenographer
(and not the jury) is your audience, you will be addressing him or
her in slow, clear careful speech that may be more formal, more
technical, and far less friendly and instructional than it would to a
jury. That is as it should be.

Clearing enough time for the deposition so that you are neither
pressured nor distracted by external commitments or deadlines is
important. Your attitude should convey, "I can continue until mid-
night, should that become necessary." This position of timeless
patience puts the onus appropriately on the attorney to move
things along.

A situation that, fortunately, occurs rarely may throw the novice
witness: a roaring fight between attorneys. The two sides, hereto-
fore quiet and almost appearing bored by the proceedings, scream

at each other, stand up in their chairs, threaten to go before the judge to plead their points, and demonstrate other regressive behavior. In one deposition, an attorney became so enraged that he stood up and threw his pen violently on the table so that bits of plastic flew into the faces of the other attorneys. Clinicians may be tempted to call on their clinical skills to temper violence, mediate the debate, or facilitate calm negotiation. Do not do anything; you will make it worse. This fight is an attorney-to-attorney matter, authentic or merely theatrical; stay seated and keep quiet until it is over. When everyone is through, the next question will be coming your way.

Assumptions. The deposing attorney may ask, "Did you make any assumptions about the case before you began?" You may be tempted to say, "Well, I know that's a good hospital, so I assumed that they knew what they were doing." This assumption is dangerous because it suggests bias, no matter how generic or basic it may seem. There are good hospitals out there, and you might well know some of them, but your belief might interfere with your detection of negligence in this case. The only assumption you should make is "good faith," meaning that you assume that the documents are what they seem to be, the parties are really the parties in the case, and so on. If the admission note turns out to be a forgery, that is not your problem; you assumed it was a medical record in good faith.

Learned treatises. In the course of a deposition, the examining attorney may ask you if a specific text (book, chapter, or article) is authoritative in the field or in the subject of the current case. Alternatively, you may be asked to supply the names of authoritative texts yourself. You then may be asked about disagreements or conflicts between your testimony and the principles stated in the text.

Most modern books and articles have multiple authors or editors; inescapably, then, these publications are not uniform in authoritativeness. However, you cannot take the position that no text is authoritative. Acknowledge that the *Comprehensive Textbook of Psychiatry* (3) has many authoritative entries, but ask to be shown to which one the attorney is referring. After reading the entry carefully, note whether you agree or disagree in general with the stated points. Remember, no one wrote a previously published book or article with the exact case in mind in which you are involved.

Attorneys tend to use the latest editions of the *Physicians' Desk Reference* (PDR) and *Diagnostic and Statistical Manual of Mental Disorders* (DSM) in a markedly concrete and reified manner. In one sense, both sources are "authoritative": PDR contains the actual package insert information about drugs, and DSM gives the formal criteria for diagnoses. But both, of course, have their limits. For example, PDR entries for the most widely used antimanic anticonvulsants may not include information about that specific usage; this is a matter of risk management for the pharmaceutical companies. Comparably, to make an informal clinical diagnosis, one may suspect a disorder based on a patient's meeting too few DSM criteria to justify a formal diagnosis, yet the clinical diagnosis and treatment still may meet the standard of care.

Novice experts, desperate for stable islands of consensus in the tossing seas of uncertainty, may imitate the attorneys by overvaluing these texts and ignoring their limits. Be sure to maintain a sense of proportion about these references and their utility.

The following excerpt cautions psychiatrists about the accuracy of testimony regarding the professional literature:

> When quoting the literature, be balanced and accurate. Give both (or several) points of view if they exist. . . . A good rule to work by is that the statements you make in court should be of the same quality and reflect the same scholarship as if you were making them at a scientific seminar or publishing them in a reputable journal. (4, p. 571)

Final predeposition preparations. Before the actual deposition, you will need to review a wide array of information. Obviously, review your files as diligently as if you were going to trial. In addition, it is wise to review—and if necessary, rehearse—the details of the links between your conclusions and the facts, statements, record notes, police reports, laboratory values, and so on so that you can buttress all your conclusions with specific elements from the database. Also, check the accuracy of any numbers (5).

In some cases, actually visiting a site may be important. Arrange to do so with the attorney sufficiently early, well before the deposition.

Meet with the attorney and review the issues. Under some circumstances, you also may want to meet one more time with the attorney's client before the deposition, especially if details remain unclear. You must exercise some care in these discussions as they may be discoverable. If you are really unsure about something, consult your own attorney; this conversation is protected. Your attorney then can communicate with the retaining attorney.

Have your attorney review your case file for any items that might be considered work product and thus under a privilege. Many attorneys anticipate this problem and send only bland correspondence; some discuss details of trial strategy in their letters to you. The latter may be privileged, but this is not your problem. Frankly admit if anything has been removed from your file; let the attorneys determine whether it is discoverable. Any notes, summaries, or "cheat sheets" (that is, outlines or summaries for quick reference) may be subject to subpoena for the deposition, and you may have to furnish copies to opposing counsel.

Above all, remember to go to bed early.

References

1. Baker TO: Operator's Manual for a Witness Chair. Milwaukee, WI, Defense Research Institute, 1983
2. Gutheil TG, Mills MJ: Legal conceptualization, legal fictions, and the manipulation of reality: conflict between models of decision-making in psychiatry and law. Bull Am Acad Psychiatry Law 10:17–27, 1982
3. Kaplan HI, Sadock BJ (eds): Comprehensive Textbook of Psychiatry/VI, 6th Edition, Vols. 1 and 2. Baltimore, MD, Willliams & Wilkins, 1995
4. Oates RK: Three do's and three don'ts for expert witnesses (editorial). Child Abuse Negl 17:571–572, 1993

5. Malone DM, Hoffman PT: The Effective Deposition: Techniques and Strategies That Work. South Bend, IN, National Institute for Trial Advocacy, 1996

Suggested Readings

Harrel PA: A new lawyer's guide to expert use: prepare your expert so you don't have to prepare for disaster. The Practical Lawyer 39:55–63, 1993

Linder RK: Preparing expert witnesses for hard questions at deposition. Defense Counsel Journal 4:174–179, 1991

Suplee DR, Woodruff MS: Deposing experts. The Practical Lawyer 33: 69–78, 1987

Suplee DR, Woodruff MS: The pretrial use of experts. The Practical Lawyer 33:9–24, 1987

6

The Expert
in Trial

Because about only 6% of all cases ever go to court—the rest are dismissed, settled, pled out, or otherwise resolved—the amount of trial time that an expert witness usually spends is often overrated by other clinicians and the public. Nevertheless, trials do come around every so often, and they are the subject of this chapter.

For experts who have spent little or no time in court, examining the companion volume, *The Psychiatrist in Court: A Survival Guide,* is recommended as an orientation. In this chapter, I review some of the basic courtroom procedures. If you are testifying away from home, be sure to review Chapter 10 in this volume before setting out.

Trial Preparation

In Chapter 6 of *The Psychiatrist in Court: A Survival Guide,* I addressed the six Ps of trial preparation. If you are uncertain about the guidelines for trial preparation, review that chapter. For the expert witness, the same six Ps should be reviewed but with a slightly different emphasis.

1. *Preparation.*   For the expert, preparation means not only reviewing the entire database with great care but also thinking through the story you plan to tell by means of your direct testimony; reviewing and analyzing opposing expert testimony and planning responses or rebuttal; and devising means of locating key passages in the database quickly.
2. *Planning.*   The importance of clearing your schedule and arranging coverage and postponement of commitments cannot be overemphasized. You do not need additional worries about what is going on at the office to cloud your focus and split your concentration. Never assume that your testimony at the trial will necessarily be over on the same day that you are scheduled to arrive for court. Build in contingency plans for the possibility that the trial extends into the next day at least. Even more distressing, some attorneys for the other side have been known to stall or drag out their questioning of you for the explicit purpose of rattling you with the need to make stay-over arrangements.

    Clarify and confirm your travel arrangements, the location of the trial, the floor of the courthouse on which the courtroom is located, parking arrangements, and all such details. Consider taking a taxicab to local courts to avoid parking hassles. If you have a disability, explore well in advance access to the courthouse and rest rooms with your attorney or with the clerk or bailiff of the court.
3. *Practice.*   You should rehearse ways of expressing information to the jury, practice sketching any visual aids you will need for the courtroom blackboard, and select useful exam-

ples from your experience to make central points. It is not enough to know the database; you need to know through choice and practice how you will convey your opinion to the jury.

4. *Pretrial conference.*   The pretrial conference is probably one of the most important stages of preparation for trial. *Insist* on this conference if the attorney is equivocal or resistant to the idea. You at least need to hear the questions that the attorney plans to ask you and to think about your answers. You also need to hear how the trial is going, what previous testimony has been given, what the judge is like, and what the emotional climate of the courtroom is. On cross-examination, if asked whether you talked to the lawyer (a query often phrased to suggest that you were coached as to your opinion), admit frankly that you insist on pretrial conferences as an essential part of preparing for your witness function.

5. *Pitfalls.*   Review the weaknesses in your opinion, the contradictory evidence, and the expected cross-examination. Clarify in your own mind how you plan to deal with questions about your fees, your publications (especially those relevant to this case), and your past experiences. Define the limits of your testimony, the unknown issues, the relevant literature, and the data relevant to the other side of the case.

6. *Presentation.*   Think about how to express your opinion and how to explain and buttress your reasoning with facts from the case. Choose some likely analogies or metaphors (discussed later in this chapter) to illustrate your points.

Practical Matters

Preparing to Go On

Many courts sequester witnesses, particularly experts; that is, experts are not allowed to be present in court for the testimony of any other witnesses. When you are allowed to hear the testimony of other witnesses, much valuable information can be gained and the tone of the room determined. Before going into the courtroom, you will find it valuable to locate the rest rooms and telephones, which are sometimes in obscure locations in older courthouses.

Once in the courtroom, rise for the judge's entrance. It is a mark of respect in many jurisdictions to rise for the jury's entrance as well, but if you are the only one standing, sit down. Wait in the public seats until actually called to the stand. Some judges take offense if they find you perched cheerfully in the witness chair before they have entered and ready to testify before being given the go-ahead to the proceedings. Some scholars recommend coming in early or during a lunch break when the court is empty to sit in the chair before you actually go on. Doing so is supposed to decrease anxiety and give you a feel for the setting (that is, where the jury will be and what the room looks like from the hot seat). Note that anxiety is normal, even for experienced experts.

What to Bring

Experts and their retaining attorneys vary in whether they prefer while testifying to have on the witness stand the entire stack of documents pertinent to the case or whether they prefer to have nothing on the stand or almost nothing (for example, only a copy of the expert report that is already in evidence or only a curriculum vitae). Each preference has its pros and cons. Recall that in almost every case, the entire database is usually present at the attorneys' tables and therefore is immediately available.

When no documents are on the stand, the opposing attorney cannot search through them for something with which to impeach your testimony. The expert is not peeking out from a daunting mound of paperwork and can face the jury directly with an unimpeded view. The expert appears more confident and knowledgeable about the case, because his or her opinion is being given from memory, as is all the substantiating data. The downside is the need to remember a vast amount of detail and to recall where, in an often extensive chart or deposition, a particular citation is. Groping for such data in the cross-examining attorney's unmarked chart—or merely recalling incorrect data—can seriously weaken your credibility.

Having the whole database on the stand permits greater support of your testimony with specific data from the documents, allows you to read the full context from which the cross-examiner may have extracted a misleading snippet, and ensures the accuracy of your recollection by direct verification. These goals are usually achieved or facilitated by some sort of quick-reference system such as highlighted text, dog-eared pages, tabs, yellow self-stick notes, or your own table of contents devised for more extensive documents. Note again the importance of having and practicing a plan of organization.

Downsides to having the entire database on the witness stand include the following: 1) you may have to lug vast tomes into court, 2) you may provide an opportunity for the cross-examiner to rummage through your files (although the effectiveness of this procedure is seriously undermined by the fact that it inevitably puts the jury to sleep and may alienate them), and 3) you may become lost in excessive data.

The expert should determine which of these two approaches is more suitable. My preference is to have only key documents on the witness stand (you almost never need to have the original complaint on the stand; if needed, the attorneys will have it). Key documents might include my report and interview notes, essential medical records (pruned to relevant periods if needed), depositions, affidavits, and similar data. It is important to include material that supports the other side of the case so as not to produce (or seem to produce) a partisan trial database. For depositions of less central players in the case, I take to the stand a one-page table of contents (that is, a list of pages on which important points are made and the gist of those points) generated earlier when I reviewed the depositions. This table of contents enables speedy reference to key facts. If I need the actual page or quote, I can use my table together with the attorney's copy of the deposition.

A handy pen or pencil, highlighting marker, and scratch pad allow you to jot unobtrusively those relevant thoughts that occur to you during your direct or cross-examination.

Finally, testifying is thirst-provoking work. Arranging for a cup, glass, or carafe of water is an excellent idea; the bailiff usually will keep it filled. A cough drop or throat lozenge will moisten your mouth while placing less of a burden on your bladder but may create a speech impediment.

What to Wear

Experts tend to fall into two general categories: 1) those who try to look like lawyers and 2) those who try to look different. It is unclear whether either strategy is superior to the other; perhaps comfort should rule. Regardless of whether you favor the charcoal pinstripe suit or the sport coat with slacks or skirt, your mode of dress should convey the fact that you are a professional in the courtroom on business. Avoid ostentation, ornamentation, eccentricity, and cutting-edge high-drama fashion or excessive informality. Stick to the conservative business mien, and you will not go wrong. Above all, do not wear new clothes; what you wear should fit well and be well broken in.

Do *not* wear or carry your cellular telephone or beeper, or if you must, ensure that they are turned off. Arrange appropriate coverage so that you do not have to worry about being reached, and check in, if you must, during breaks. Judges and juries find the shrill sound of the beeper intrusive and annoying and interpret it as arrogance, showing off how busy you are and how court is taking you away from really important matters. Indeed, some judges get quite exercised and sarcastic when paging intrudes on the court sanctum.

If you are completely uncertain about what to wear to court, see also "Dressing for Success" in Chapter 6 in *The Psychiatrist in Court: A Survival Guide.*

Demeanor

Being on the stand is not unlike being filmed, in the sense that you are usually under observation by someone at all times, even when someone else is speaking: the bailiff, the bored juror, the defendant or plaintiff, an attorney. Avoid personal body attentions (such as scratching) as much as possible. Beware of "involuntary" gestures, such as rolling your eyes at the jury when a particularly fatuous question is asked. Such reactions may be misconstrued as disrespectful, not of the attorney in question but of the jury or the entire process. Scholars recommend keeping the front of your body open (for example, by not folding your arms) as body language consistent with candor. Find a relaxed but alert position on the stand and settle into it to avoid shifting or squirming.

Your identity on the stand is that of teacher. Be clear; get interested in what you have to say and stay interested. Make your point because it matters, it is important, and you *want* the jury to understand it. An expert who doesn't seem to care about his or her own testimony has probably irreversibly lost the jury: why should they care if the expert doesn't?

Humor usually is a valuable teaching tool; however, in court it should be treated as a double-edged weapon likely to turn and cut the wielder. This unpredictability flows from the fact that you are not sure of an emotional alliance with the jury at all points along the way. Without such alliance, humor may seem disrespectful, flip, obnoxiously facetious, or obtuse to the seriousness of the issue, as the opposing lawyer will immediately try to point out. With discretion, humor directed against yourself may show that you do not take yourself too seriously. A colleague reported the following:

> *Attorney:* What is your academic rank at Harvard Medical
> School?
> *Witness:* I am an instructor in psychiatry at Harvard.
> *Attorney (with a slight sneer):* Isn't it true, Doctor, that
> instructor is the lowest rank in the academic system
> there?
> *Witness:* You sure know how to hurt a guy [general
> laughter; attorney moves on to another subject].

Three common demeanor pitfalls for the expert that negatively impinge on credibility are being huffy, fluffy, and stuffy.

There is no reason for a teacher to get mad. Even when an attorney attacks you, demeans you, impugns you, or degrades you, you know or should know that it is not personal and has nothing to do with you. If the attorney is hostile, sneering, and sarcastic, and you are unfailingly polite, you win. If you become huffy or outright mad, you are likely to be too involved and therefore possibly biased, not credible. A witness with an apparent chip on his or her shoulder (and in court, all such chips are apparent) is particularly unconvincing.

Being fluffy means being too abstract, theoretical, jargon laden, evasive, and "waffley." Make your point as concretely as necessary and back it up with hard data from the database. If you must use, explain, or respond to jargon, adopt a self-deprecating or ironic attitude toward it that includes the jury in an alliance (that is, what fools these jargonists be). In general, avoid discussing unconscious dynamics unless absolutely needed for your point; they are usually poorly received by juries.

Finally, good teachers are lively and interesting, not stuffy. They are not excessively academic, pedantic, or prone to nit-picking. Haggling with the attorney over a tiny abstruse point, or waxing argumentative rather than instructive, blunts your argument and weakens your credibility; concede a remote possibility and move on. As occurs during the deposition, the most common beginner's error in the courtroom is the inability to "throw it away," that is, to concede a point that really doesn't mean much, to accept a possibility as such (anything is "possible," but only a few things reach reasonable medical certainty), to agree that some things happen sometimes, and to admit that rules have exceptions.

Remember that "reasonable medical certainty" is a standard of testimony that connotes "more likely than not"; the concept is sometimes rendered mathematically as a 51% certainty. Because jurisdictions differ as to the precise definition, the expert should find out the relevant local standard and employ it (see also Chapter 6 in *The Psychiatrist in Court: A Survival Guide*).

Testimony

Direct testimony should unfold in an organized manner, as a result of your careful and thoughtful preparation with your attorney. Direct your extended remarks to the jury, making eye contact whenever possible. Speak to the most distant juror to be sure your voice is audible; a jury that cannot hear may be hesitant about saying so in open court yet may ultimately give up on you after straining to hear for too long. If a microphone is available, adjust its distance from your face to minimize annoying popping noises on plosives such as *b* and *p*. If no microphone is provided, project. If in any doubt about your speech volume, ask if you can be heard by the farthest ranks of jurors; even inhibited souls will nod if they can hear.

Keep in mind the expert's role in telling the story in a coherent, understandable manner that brings the details together in a recognizable gestalt. Although you are a teacher, the trial is a human process, not just a classroom exercise.

Remember that no matter how intensely you may feel about anything, you must scrupulously avoid any of the mildest forms of profanity or blasphemy, even as rhetorical devices. In some parts of the country, and for some jurors, saying "Lord, no!" for emphasis in answer to a question involves breaking one of the Ten Commandments.

There are various reasons for the expert to use a blackboard, marker board, or flip chart (for further discussion, see Chapter 6 in *The Psychiatrist in Court: A Survival Guide*). The expert should prepare some information that can be presented effectively by using one of these aids, if only to break the talking-heads monotony of witness after witness. Make sure you can be heard when using the blackboard, marker board, or flip chart because if there is a microphone, you will now be away from it. Do not be ashamed to boom it out. Similarly, be sure to write large enough to be read by the *farthest* juror; ask the far ranks if they can see the first letter or picture you write or draw. If not, increase the scale. Novice experts may not be aware that the witness who faces the blackboard and mumbles the sound-track accompaniment to his micrographia is not only ineffective but also actively alienating, possibly even insulting, the jury.

When responding to cross-examination, maintain the identical level of interest, animation, politeness, and responsiveness as you demonstrated on direct examination (although you are allowed to become more alert). The expert who is warm, winning, and discursive on direct examination only to turn crabbed, argumentative, defensive, and guarded on cross-examination is communicating only bias. You are telling the truth; what difference does it make which side is asking the questions? The hostile, attacking attorney who meets with your unfailing politeness and persistent civility is perpetrating suicide, not homicide. If either side asks a genuinely excellent question, say so but only if you mean it.

Answering cross-examination questions does not require that you help out the attorney with various possible misunderstandings he or she may have about psychiatry; just answer the question. The only exception to this rule is when so profound a misunderstanding of some fact is taking place that for you to answer the question would merely precipitate and perpetuate a French farce situation of two parties on totally different wavelengths; this situation is not funny in court. Clarify the point, then wait for the next question.

Some Pointers

Some experts develop a code with their attorney to aid covering certain points brought out on cross-examination. For example, expert and attorney may agree that if the expert prefaces an answer on cross-examination with, "Well, that's an interesting point, . . . " it means that the expert wishes to be asked about the issue on redirect. Such an arrangement may be considered, but in practice it may be more cumbersome and distracting than it is worth.

In a personal communication (K. Lipez, November 1996), an experienced judge noted that his opinion of an expert falls if the expert has failed to anticipate, and seems unprepared for, an obvious line of questioning. For example, in a criminal trial with a proposed insanity defense, the question of malingering is highly relevant. An expert who seems surprised at this issue being brought out on cross-examination reveals serious lacunae in understanding the forensic issues involved.

The same judge cautioned against too facile a psychiatric or psychological explanation of human behavior. The posture that everything can be explained (or even worse, "*I* can explain everything") is unconvincing to juries and may even imply that the patient has succeeded in manipulating the psychiatrist.

Finally, I suggest giving up the fantasy of being able to predict entirely the effect of what you say on the jury: the jury will decide how the jury will decide. In a case in which a psychiatrist was being sued for malpractice in a patient's suicide, I gave extensive defense testimony and remarked, strictly in passing, that although it would not be ethical to give my own independent diagnosis—because I had not seen the patient—the diagnosis given by those who had seen the patient was fully consistent with the recorded symptoms. A poll of the jury after the defense verdict revealed that the jury had been impressed and perhaps even swayed by the fact that the only witnesses who used the word *ethical* were I and the physician-defendant.

An especially sticky and dismaying problem, fortunately not that common, is the situation wherein the attorney has misunderstood some fundamental clinical issue, and neither he or she nor you has realized that this misunderstanding exists. I was testifying for the defense before a licensing board in a sexual misconduct complaint. In the middle of direct examination, the attorney developed a line of questioning, with which I was implicitly asked to agree, that appeared based on the theory that because the patient (whom I hadn't seen) evinced borderline personality disorder (BPD) the claim was likely to be false. (This conclusion represents an unfortunate misperception of the findings in an article of mine [1]. In fact, given the actual frequency of sexual misconduct complaints by BPD patients against their therapists, patients with BPD are statistically more likely to be initiators of true claims than false ones.) Horrified at this evolving debacle and unable to stop it or even comment on it until the next break, I took refuge where all witnesses in such a spot should take it: the absolute truth. The attorney might catch on or might not, might be baffled or might not, might be annoyed with you afterward or might not, but those are not your problems. The oath always provides sanctuary in a storm.

A similar dilemma faces the testifying expert when some significant fact is revealed for the first time during trial testimony—a fact that changes your opinion. Do not panic and feel guilty, abashed, or inadequate. This revelation may be the lawyer's lapse, but it is not your problem. Your job is to tell the truth; if the facts substantively change, an ethical expert's opinion would be expected to change.

Language Level

Remember to keep your testimony basic and jargon free. Illustrate your points with analogies and metaphors that you believe the average jury will follow. The following is an example of how you might discuss the mechanism of action of a selective serotonin reuptake inhibitor:

> You know that the spark plugs on your car work by sending a spark across a narrow gap (show by using your fingers). Well, the nerves in your nervous system, including the nerves that control your mood, communicate in the same way (sketch a synapse). The upstream nerve sends an electrical current (draw a lightning bolt) down to this spark gap called a synapse (write word on board), and when it gets there, the current releases little blobs of chemicals like tiny water balloons. These float across the spark gap and hit certain "hot buttons" on the end of the downstream nerve and set off the next electrical current (draw another lightning bolt). Now that these chemicals are out there, how do you turn them off for the next bolt? The upstream nerve sucks them back up like a vacuum cleaner, and the system is ready for the next nerve impulse. Now this medication blocks (draw a barrier) this process, just like putting your hand over the vacuum nozzle; if you do that, the dirt stays on the floor. In the same way, the chemicals stay in the spark gap and keep working so that your mood is lifted. That is how this kind of antidepressant or mood elevator works.

Although this mode of explanation may seem cumbersome, the jury usually appreciates being given the "inside story," but this appreciation is lost if the jury cannot understand or follow your description. Consider practicing such a description with your attorney or colleagues or friends.

The hazards of lack of practice are revealed by this following segment from an actual murder trial. The expert is on direct examination by his retaining attorney.

> Um—he went—um—a couple of days after that to the—um—[mental health center]—um—and—um—complaining of feeling stressed, depressed—um—and seeking help. Um—as the events became closer to the—um—incident itself [the murder],—um— I think that—um—[defendant] was—um—was very upset by the scene on [date] in which he observed his wife.

As you can grasp by merely reading this response aloud, it is numbing to a jury. Recall that this is direct examination by his *own* retaining attorney, and the expert has theoretically prepared to tell the story in a coherent manner. What will cross-examination be like? What is the jury to make of this apparent hesitancy and doubt?

Remember also that the court reporter slavishly but perfectly appropriately records every pause, stutter, and throat clear that you emit on the stand. This is a powerful argument for at least organizing your thoughts before you begin to testify.

Respect the juror; do not underestimate juries. Over the years, I have been impressed by their ability to grasp what is at issue, even if the technical details are lost in the shuffle. Respect their native intelligence by preparing clear ways of communicating the bases for your opinions.

Adventures in Cross-Examination

For experienced experts, some scholars assert, the best cross-examination is, "I have no questions for this witness," preferably said in a mildly contemptuous tone, as if to convey, "I don't care to waste my time on this whore; any testimony from *this* witness would be bought and meaningless." Realistically, such an avoidance of cross-examination is sound trial strategy, because a seasoned expert will simply use cross-examination as an opportunity to make some of the same points made on direct with different emphases. The jury hears the testimony twice—an aid to both memory and persuasion.

Most often, however, attorneys do not perform this simple but effective maneuver. Attorneys will not avoid cross-examining the expert for several reasons: the attorney's narcissism ("I can handle this expert on cross-examination, no problem.") or exhibitionism ("Watch me shine!"); the attorney's wish or need to have the client see the attorney doing something, as opposed to the attorney's apparently doing nothing (clients often do not grasp the power of "I have no questions"); the attorney's competitive strivings with the opposing attorney or firm; and even the attorney's competitive feelings directed toward the expert.

Even those attorneys who opt to engage in cross-examination are usually (but, surprisingly, not always) aware of two fundamental principles that guide this activity. First, never ask a question to which you do not already know the answer, or alternatively, ask only questions to which only one answer is possible (fittingly, questions beginning "Is it possible . . . " are almost always answered yes on the theory that anything is possible). The attorney may know the answer to a particular question from the expert's report, interrogatory, deposition, or publications, or the answer may be obvious from the question (that is, the question answers itself). Some examples of the latter follow (all are leading questions, which may be asked on cross- but not on direct examination):

- "Isn't it true that a patient's condition can sometimes change rapidly in a short time?"
- "Psychiatrists can be fooled about a patient's sanity, can they not?"
- "Another expert might come to a different conclusion, isn't that right, Doctor?"

The only possible truthful answer to all the aforementioned questions is yes. Throw it away; equivocating hurts you.

The second fundamental principle of expert cross-examination is keep the expert on a tight rein. The attorney avoids asking open-ended questions that permit the expert to repeat or expand on direct testimony. Instead, the attorney asks closed questions, such as the previously listed leading questions.

The tight rein on which you are held may make it difficult to get your opinion out there. Experienced experts sometimes begin their responses with the subordinate clause rather than the main one, forcing the cross-examining attorney to permit them to finish their statements rather than cutting them off. If you want to say, "that's generally true, but in this instance it is not," the attorney may move on to the next question after you have said, "that's generally true" and you may be too flustered to challenge the action. It is better to say, "Although the present case is a clear exception to that rule, what you say is often true in other cases."

The tyranny of yes or no.   You will be on the shortest rein when the attorney uses the most closed format of questioning—the one demanding that you answer only yes or no. Practically, this type of questioning means that you have only three answers available: "yes," "no," and "that question cannot truthfully be answered yes or no." The key word is *truthfully.* You took an oath to tell the whole truth, and a mere yes or no may fail to convey the "whole truth." Listen with intense attention to the question, and think seriously about whether yes or no will represent the whole truth. If either will do so, say it; if not, state that you cannot answer yes or no.

Quotes.   On cross-examination, the attorney may quote something that you wrote or lectured on. Always ask to see the context if you do not immediately and completely recall it because removing a remark from its original context is a common mechanism attorneys use to impeach you with your own words. Remember that you did not write the article or make the statement during a lecture with this particular case in mind.

After Rodin.   Pause briefly before answering each question to allow replay of the query in your mind, to be sure you are clear about the question, to consider your answer carefully, and to allow your attorney to object, if needed. At times, a question will require more time for prolonged thought or searching of your memory. Your thinking in silence may confuse the jury: are you paralyzed with dismay at the cross-examination, or have you dozed off? It is best to state, "I'm going to take a moment to think about that," and do so. I seriously recommend that you try to look as if you are thinking to clarify for the jury what this pause in the proceedings is all about and to allow those *jurors* who have dozed off to be awakened by the sudden silence. At such moments, a judge may even decide to declare a recess: "While you are thinking, Doctor, we are going to take our midmorning break right now. We'll reconvene in 15 minutes." The break gives you ample time to think.

Breaks.   During breaks that occur in the middle of cross-examination, some attorneys advise not discussing your testimony, because "What did you discuss?" may well be the first question when you are back on the stand (only discussions with your own lawyer are protected). Some experts want to call their offices during breaks; others find telephone calls distracting and let whoever is covering for them handle things.

For the lunch break, I recommend avoiding eating heavily. Some experts have only an iced tea for lunch and forgo any other intake to avoid postprandial torpor and the dulling of attention that may accompany it. Use your own judgment and knowledge of your biorhythms.

The final opinion.   During the course of expert consultation, you may have written a report after reviewing some quantity of material. Later, you may have been deposed, and some additional material may have come your way just before the trial (which, had it changed your opinion, you would have been obligated to so inform your attorney, but let's assume it did not). Now you must testify on the witness stand.

The cross-examining attorney may make an issue of the fact that you had not seen a particular document or known a particular fact before you gave your opinions in your report or deposition. The thrust of this line of questioning is to convey that your opinion is premature, incomplete, or inadequately grounded in data. Remember that your opinion is steadily evolving as increments of material are conveyed to you and as your analysis proceeds.

Your *final* opinion, the one that counts, is your actual trial testimony. In theory, your opinion, because it is based on data, could change with complete validity based on some new fact that you hear for the first time during the trial. This change is as it should be. If your opinion does *not* change under these circumstances of a novel and significant contradiction of previous data, you have confused loyalty to your attorney with the oath to tell the truth.

An aid to this conceptualization is to label your first report, if requested, as a preliminary report. Subsequent communications may be labeled supplementary reports to keep the sequence clear.

Crises

Various crises may strike while you are on the stand. These include biological and physiological crises or circumstantial ones, such as the discovery that you have left a key document in your suitcase across the courtroom.

Do not hesitate to ask the judge to permit you to take a break for these reasons. Do not be inhibited by fears that, by needing to go to the bathroom, for example, you will appear inept, entitled, childish, sickly, or weak. Your job as expert is important to the case, and serious distractions impair your work. Deal with the problem and then continue with your task with restored focus.

It is probably inappropriate to ask for a break only because the cross-examination is strenuous and effective and you wish to break the flow. Your attorney may recognize the problem and ask for a sidebar conference or other delaying tactic. If a delaying tactic is not used, it is preferable just to hang in there. Use breaks or the jury's distraction by the attorneys' wrangling as an opportunity to wipe sweat discreetly from your brow. Focus on slow, measured breathing; stretch your limbs behind the screen of the stand; and sit more upright to relieve tension.

The End of the Affair

Finally, the seemingly interminable re-re-redirect and re-re-recross-examination have worn the two attorneys into a torpor, and both grudgingly acknowledge that neither has any more questions for you. The judge dismisses you by saying, "You (or the witness) may step down" or "Thank you, Doctor, that's all."

At this point you say, "Thank you, Your Honor," pack up your papers (being careful not to include and therefore abscond with any official case exhibits), get down from the stand, nod politely to the jury, and go. Some more extroverted experts thank the jury out loud, wave at the jury box ("So long, fans!"), or emit other social behaviors. No one knows the effect of these gestures; as always, conservativeness is probably better (the discreet nod rather than the glad-hand wave).

Forensic etiquette requires that you just leave. Do not stop to chat or debrief with the attorney. Do not hang around to hear what other witnesses say, to see the outcome, or to learn of other subsequent activity. This behavior conveys too much interest in the outcome for someone who is not a party to the case. What do you care what happens? You only testify under oath; when you are through, you exit.

If you have traveled far with a heavy load of database materials, consider making advance arrangements with the attorney so that he or she will hold on to your case materials and retain or discard them as desired. Take only your report.

Most courteous attorneys will inform you later, by letter or telephone, as much as possible about what happened and why it happened. Some forget. It is perfectly appropriate after some time has passed to call and ask the outcome. For your personal development as an expert, always seek feedback and reactions.

Finally, I recommend against keeping a won-lost record of how the trial went according to the side for which you testified; this task is for the lawyers. Forces beyond your control and outside your testimony impinge on trial outcome. I recommend instead treating each testimony experience as a kind of continuing education: What did you learn? What questions were you asked that caught you by surprise? Which crafty attorney's gambits succeeded and which failed during your cross-examination? Did you in fact get to make the points that you believe needed to be made? Did you feel you were clear to the jury? Was there a better way of explaining or describing something other than the way it came out in court? These questions and their thoughtful answers are the true indexes of your success in trial.

Reference

1. Gutheil TG: Borderline personality disorder, boundary violations and patient-therapist sex: medicolegal pitfalls. Am J Psychiatry 146:597–602, 1989

Suggested Readings

Appelbaum PS: Evaluating the admissibility of expert testimony. Hosp Community Psychiatry 45:9–10, 1994

Goldstein RL: Psychiatrists in the hot seat: discrediting doctors by impeachment of their credibility. Bull Am Acad Psychiatry Law 16: 225–234, 1988

Hollander N, Baldwin LM: Winning with experts. Trial 1:16–24, 1992

Langerman AG: Making sure your experts shine: effective presentation of expert witnesses. Trial 1:106–110, 1992

Lubet S: Effective use of experts: eight techniques for the direct examination of experts. Trial 2:16–20, 1993

McIntyre MA: Use and abuse of articles and publications in cross-examining an expert witness. Trial 2:23–24, 1993

Moore TA: Medical negligence: cross-examining the defense expert. Trial 1:49–52, 1991

Shuman DW: Psychiatric and Psychological Evidence. Colorado Springs, CO, Shepard's/McGraw-Hill, 1988

Suplee DR, Woodruff MS: Cross examination of expert witnesses. The Practical Lawyer 34:41–54, 1987a

Suplee DR, Woodruff MS: Direct examination of experts. The Practical Lawyer 33:53–60, 1987b

Wawro MLD: Effective presentation of experts. Litigation 19:31–37, 1993

7

Some Pointers on Expert Witness Practice

In this chapter, I address some practical issues about being an expert witness. Some of the points covered are received wisdom; others flow empirically from experience. The aim is to help you meet the challenges along the way.

Scheduling Issues

One of the most challenging and complex problems that the expert witness faces is the matter of scheduling time in general and trial time in particular. General time constraints require you to plan creatively for the blocks of your schedule that will be occupied by

your case review. Similarly, you will be trying to fit your other forensic activities (review, depositions, trial) into the interstices of
your clinical or administrative work.

Always remember that the fundamental rhythm of the trial is
"hurry up and wait." If you cannot stand reviewing the case any-
more lest you explode, read something else. Keep a paperback or
journal handy for filling voids.

Priorities

It is every expert's nightmare that several commitments will con-
verge on the same tiny allocation of time. In accordance with Mur-
phy's Law, you will go for months without any forensic activity
whatsoever, but during the very week that you have scheduled four
weddings and a funeral, two trials in different states will be called
simultaneously, with a deposition for a third case. This type of
schedule is reality.

Such a conjunction of scheduling conflicts requires a great deal
of diplomacy, negotiation, and telephone calls to resolve them. As
a rule of thumb, the hierarchy of urgency and therefore attempted
postponement (or at worst, cancellation) is as follows.

Trials take first priority. Large numbers of people are involved,
court dockets are crowded and leave little flexibility, and serious
matters hang in the balance. You may have a little room to maneuver in terms of the order in which you testify. An attorney who
planned to have you "bat cleanup" (that is, testify last in order to
summarize) may be willing to move you earlier in the case and
somewhat restructure your direct examination to compensate for
this maneuver. In extreme circumstances, the other side may be
willing to have your testimony inserted into their side of the case,
with suitable preparation of the jury.

The tension here is that some courts, attorneys, and other-side
attorneys are reasonable, flexible, and accommodating; others are
not. You must do the best you can with what you've got. Because
your attorney has the most interest in your presence, he or she

will be exerting the greatest efforts to make it all work out, but things happen. Travel glitches (discussed in Chapter 10 in this volume), of course, add another layer of challenge.

The second priority is depositions, which also require several people to synchronize their schedules, although obviously fewer persons and a shorter time frame are involved than are for trial. If a trial and a deposition are scheduled for the same time, the trial should take precedence.

The last two priorities are interview and report. Because your reports can be done at any time of the day or night, theoretically, a forensic interview, requiring two parties to match schedules, comes before a report.

Trial Time Considerations

A cheerful bit of dialogue that experts hear constantly is, for example: "Doctor, I know you have a busy schedule, so let's put you on first at 9:00 A.M. sharp. I can't imagine my direct examination taking more than an hour, tops. You'll probably be cross-examined for 1, maybe 2, hours. You'll be out of there by lunchtime."

Smile politely when you hear these words but make expansive plans. You can count on your eyeballs the number of times this clockwork model actually occurs. Why? Although some judges are scrupulously punctual, some are not. Occasionally, a judge will treat the time between 9:00 and 9:30 A.M. as a kind of swing time in which he or she can hear a half dozen motions in this and other cases and "dispose of them." In addition, the odd juror gets stuck in traffic. The attorneys wrangle over whether some document relevant to the next witness is admissible. The jury takes a long midmorning break. The judge assigns a long lunch and hears another few motions just afterward. Thus, it is not uncommon for an out-by-noon case to extend into the next day.

The aforementioned realities make it essential for you to clear as much time as possible for a trial appearance. (More suggestions on scheduling are included in Chapter 10 in this volume.)

Your So-Called Life

Another scheduling issue almost entirely ignored in the forensic professional literature is the question of events in your personal life that may conflict with forensic commitments. Although my colleagues and I tried to study this issue formally (1), no clear conclusions can be drawn. The subject may represent some kind of taboo because it is rarely discussed. However, negotiation may be possible for some scheduling conflicts but not always. In the end, difficult choices may have to be made. The best aid for peace of mind for the would-be forensic expert is an understanding spouse, partner, and family.

Reference

1. Kearney AJ, Gutheil TG, Commons ML: Trading forensic and family commitments. Bull Am Acad Psychiatry Law 24:533–546, 1996

Suggested Reading

Modlin HC, Felthous A: Forensic psychiatry in practice. Bull Am Acad Psychiatry Law 17:69–82, 1989

8

Writing to and for the Legal System

The expert witness may provide many different kinds of written documentation to the legal system, an attorney, a court, or a quasi-legal agency such as a board of registration or a bureau of motor vehicles. Examples of such writing include a letter providing an assessment of a person's fitness to drive, to serve as a witness, or to serve on a jury; a description of an independent medical examination for a personal injury suit, for a worker's compensation claim, or for a disability determination; or a full evaluation of a person's competence to stand trial, a defendant's criminal responsibility, or a physician's deviation from the standard of care.

In all such cases, attention to the preparation of the written document results in a product that assists the legal system in its efforts and goals and validates your contribution to the process.

In *The Psychiatrist in Court: A Survival Guide,* some basic principles on letter writing to the court are described and are not repeated in this chapter. In this chapter, I focus on writing the full-fledged forensic report.

The Forensic Report

Writing a forensic report is an important function of the expert for a number of reasons. The report may be the first time the attorney who retained you has had an opportunity to see your opinions in written form, allowing careful legal analysis and reflection on whether you will be helpful on the case. Alternatively, your report may open up entirely novel approaches to litigating the case or new issues to develop on cross-examination of the opposing experts. In other situations, your report may be the decisive factor in convincing the other side of the case to settle or drop the matter. These are all powerful arguments for careful thought, painstaking preparation, and meticulous proofing and review of any report you produce.

Despite these useful functions, the report may present materials or approaches that the attorney does not wish to share with the other side. Consequently, the attorney may ask that you not furnish a report, which in that jurisdiction is discoverable by the other side. For similar reasons, the attorney may request a bare-bones report describing only the materials that you have reviewed and your concluding opinions, without detailed discussion of the bases or reasoning behind those conclusions.

Forensic report writing, then, may take three major forms (with variations possible, of course): 1) no report, in which case you are asked to summarize your views in a nondiscoverable telephone call for the attorney's benefit; 2) a summary report, which presents your database and conclusions only; and 3) the full, detailed report, which states all of your conclusions and the analysis of all the relevant substantiating data. In this chapter, I emphasize the third form, because the first is self-explanatory and the second is an extract of the third.

Phillip J. Resnick, M.D., a leading forensic scholar who lectures on forensic report writing at the annual forensic review course of the American Academy of Psychiatry and the Law, has generously and graciously granted me permission to cite some of his advice on report writing, for which I am most grateful (where I cite his material, I refer to him explicitly in the text).

General Remarks

The report as a whole should meet certain criteria. It should contain everything that you need to support your opinion and no irrelevant material. It should be just long enough to cover the essential information but not so long as to exhaust the reader. It should stand alone. According to Dr. Resnick, "Reports should be self-sufficient. Without referring to other documents, the reader should be able to understand how the opinion was reached from the data in the report. Critical documents should be briefly summarized within the report."

Dr. Resnick also identifies the "four principles of good writing": clarity, simplicity, brevity, and humanity. Obviously, all should govern the form of the report.

The Heading

The first report should be titled "Preliminary Report," and subsequent contributions, additions, or emendations should be titled "Supplementary Report." The reasoning is that the "Final Report" would be your trial testimony itself (if the trial occurs), testimony which might theoretically be influenced by new information emerging during the trial testimony of other witnesses. The heading also might include your name and the date of the report.

Identifying data can be presented in a number of ways. One way is to provide the case citation or caption in whole or in brief (for example, *Smith v. Jones et al.* or *State v. John Johnson*), the case or docket number if known, the charges in a criminal case, or the type of case in a civil matter (for example, emotional injury or psychiatric malpractice).

Some experts and their retaining attorneys prefer that the report be in the form of a letter addressed to the attorney. In that case, use a standard business letter format; otherwise, think of your report as a memorandum and use a standardized format. One model by Dr. Resnick is included at the end of this chapter.

The Occasion

The occasion, sometimes called the referral, of the report should address the question of why you are writing this report; that is, what is your standing in the case that justifies this missive? How and why did this examinee get to your doorstep? Examples might include the following:

- "At the request of Attorney John Smith (or Judge Janet Jones), I examined (name of examinee) with regard to (forensic issue). . . . "
- "I examined Ms. Susan Smith at her own request to document her competence to make a will on the occasion of her plans to alter her bequest. . . . "

Some attorneys, reasoning that the occasion is obvious from context, may prefer that you simply plunge in:

- "In preparing this preliminary report I have reviewed the following documents, . . . "

The Database

After identifying the occasion, the report should ordinarily present a listing of everything you have reviewed in preparing the report: medical records, police reports, legal pleadings, and depositions. Include any interviews performed and their date and length. This listing is best presented in tabular fashion to allow ease of checking whether you have reviewed all relevant materials. The documents may be listed alphabetically, chronologically, or according to some natural, logical grouping (for example, all medical reports, all depositions).

The Conclusion or Opinion

The great schism between schools of forensic report writing lies between the conclusion-first advocates and conclusion-last devotees. Although each group has a rationale, no convincing case has been made for the inherent superiority of either approach; you are free to choose your favorite.

The rationale for placing the conclusion just after the database list (and thus at or near the beginning of the report) is that the reader (judge, attorney, or other) is free to stop there and make decisions about future directions in which the process should go, about the disposition, and so on. The remainder of the report is thus treated as optional reading. Such an approach appeals to busy judges who want to get to the punch line without having to listen to the long-winded joke.

The rationale for placing the conclusion last is that such a structure allows the reader to develop an evolving (and therefore deeper) sense of the expert's reasoning as it may (or may not) lead to the conclusion. The expert escapes the accusation of being too conclusive in voicing the opinion by providing the steps and stages of reasoning that point to the outcome.

It is important to couch your conclusion in the explicit jurisdiction-specific language defined in case law or statute (your lawyer should inform you what this is) and to state it according to the standard of reasonable medical certainty to render your report material and admissible. A typical conclusion in a malpractice case, for example, might take the following form:

Conclusion

Based on my review of the above materials (the database) and my own training and experience, it is my professional opinion, held to a reasonable degree of medical certainty, that, in the treatment of (plaintiff), (defendant) failed to practice at the standard of care of the average reasonable practitioner in that specialty and that stage of training . . . (or, the treatment provided to [plaintiff] by [defendant] comported well with [or within] the standard).

Note the wording. First, the overall basis is described as both the database (all the material reviewed in the case, including interview data) and total clinical background of training (what you were taught) and experience (what you have found for yourself by practicing in the field about which you are testifying). Second, you are voicing a professional opinion (rather than a casual or personal one) to a particular standard of testimony called reasonable medical certainty (that is, more likely than not). Third, you are explicitly stating your opinion in the statutory or other definition of malpractice used in that locality. Finally, you do *not* say "the defendant committed malpractice" because only the fact finder can address that ultimate issue. Your testimony is focused on and limited to the underlying criteria for the forensic determination you are making, be it competence, insanity, or malpractice.

Supporting Data

After the conclusion, you can present the supporting material in several ways. If your conclusion is stated at the outset, you may provide the supporting data in any coherent and logical manner (such as by the categories of a standard psychiatric workup or by type of data such as an interview or a deposition). Dr. Resnick suggests using subheadings to organize the information and facilitate the flow of the report.

It cannot be overemphasized how critical this phase of the report will be to the credibility and utility of your opinion. Remember that the conclusion, although representing the core of your opinion, is essentially boilerplate (that is, standardized legal language). Your ability to back up *every one* of your conclusions with multiple specific examples and corroborations from the database is the essential test of your value, effectiveness, and credibility as an expert witness.

If your conclusion comes at the end of the report, this section should contain extracts of previous material directly supporting the points you are making. Dr. Resnick explains, "Reasons supporting opinions should be clearly and fully stated. The reader should not have to use his/her own inferences to understand the point."

Multiple Realities

In civil cases, it is predictable that plaintiff and defendant tell different stories, sometimes frankly contradictory, sometimes different spins on the truth. In criminal cases involving the insanity defense, the defendant usually has admitted the act for which he or she is charged, but occasionally, a case involves the attorney's asking for a criminal responsibility assessment when the defendant denies even doing the criminal act.

In these cases, the expert should scrupulously avoid assuming one side is correct. As Dr. Resnick states, "If there are two versions of the facts, offer alternative opinions." In every case, your conclusions should be presented in the following form: "If the allegations are true, then. . . . " This approach prevents your seeming to side with one party in the case.

Constraints, Limits, and Rebuttals

If there have been any constraints of time, money, or data (such as inadmissible material, interview of plaintiff blocked by attorney, attorney will not pay for travel to see examinee) or limits imposed on the conclusions by any circumstances in the case, these should be recorded. These are not weaknesses of the report; on the contrary, it would be a weakness not to acknowledge these factors candidly.

Opinions differ on whether the expert should present overt self-rebuttal possibilities to his or her own opinions, including evidence opposing those views (even if outweighed by other evidence supporting them) or alternative conclusions derived from some of the same data. Some attorneys suggest that including points relevant to the other side of the case enhances your credibility and suggests greater objectivity, which make for a stronger report. Other attorneys feel this is unnecessary or detrimental and assert that cross-examination should be left to the cross-examiner. Whichever approach you actually take in your written report, it is essential that you identify and remain ready to testify under oath to such contradicting factors if asked under cross-examination (or direct examination for that matter).

Postreport Negotiations

After your report is finished and has been sent to the attorney, judge, or agency for which it has been prepared, you may receive requests to alter the report in some ways. Some requested alterations are fully ethical; some are not.

Ethical alterations include changing the language of your conclusions to meet precisely the statutory wording, asking for the addition of new material not supplied to you earlier, and shortening the report by aggressive editing, summarizing, and deleting. (Remember you must be candid about everything you believe to be true, even if it has been removed from your report for brevity.)

Unethical requests for alterations include asking you to reach opinions unsubstantiated by the data, to alter or misrepresent facts in the database, or to change the substance of your opinions.

A challenging gray zone is negotiating about wording. There is no absolute guideline for this procedure, but generally there is no inherent problem in adjusting wording as long as the substance of your opinion is not changed thereby. Be careful about changing wording concerning issues of causation, intensity (likely, very likely, extremely likely), and effect of emotional injuries—three common problem areas.

The Experience Factor

This chapter alone cannot prepare you fully for forensic report writing, but it may get you started. There is probably no substitute for practice and feedback from your retaining attorney and peers in the field. I strongly recommend having an experienced colleague review your early reports and offer critiques and feedback. You also may ask to see a senior colleague's report under an agreement of confidentiality.

The Criminal Report: An Example

The following is Dr. Resnick's outline for a typical criminal report.[1]

1. Identifying information:
2. Source of referral:
3. Referral issue:
4. Sources of information:
5. Qualifications of the examiner:
6. Statement of nonconfidentiality:
7. Past personal history:
8. Family history:
9. Sexual and marital history:
10. Educational history:
11. Employment history:
12. Military history:
13. Relevant medical history:
14. Drug and alcohol history:
15. Legal history:
16. Psychiatric history:
17. Prior relationship of the defendant to the victim:
18. Defendant's account of the crime:
19. Witness and/or victim accounts of the crime:
20. Mental status examination:
21. Physical examination and laboratory tests:
22. Summary of psychological testing:

---

[1]Used with permission.

23. Competency assessment:
24. Psychiatric diagnosis:
25. Opinion:

Suggested Readings

Hoffman BF: How to write a psychiatric report for litigation following a personal injury. Am J Psychiatry 143:164–169, 1986

Melton GB, Petrilla J, Poythress NG, et al (eds): Consultation, report writing and expert testimony, in Psychological Evaluations for the Courts: A Handbook for Mental Health Professionals and Lawyers, Vol 3. New York, Guilford, 1987, pp 347–371

Weiner IB: Writing forensic reports, in Handbook of Forensic Psychology. Edited by Weiner IB, Hess AK. New York, Wiley, 1987, pp 511–528

9

Developing and Marketing a Forensic Practice

How to get started in forensic work is a common preoccupation among novice expert witnesses. Unfortunately, the path to success in effectively and ethically developing and marketing a forensic practice is fraught with many false steps, embarrassments, and inefficacies. In this chapter, I describe successful strategies for developing and marketing a forensic practice as well as means of avoiding some common pitfalls.

In the late 1970s, two residency classmates and I realized that we were all getting into forensic work and decided to form a group or corporation. In addition to the (largely fantasied) corporate benefits we dreamed we would derive, such an affiliation would mean that we would be able to say to any attorney who called us, "Yes! We (or the corporation) will take your case. We will let you know shortly which of our directors will be working with you." The ability to say yes to all comers seemed like a good idea at the time.

We retained an industrial designer to help create a logo (highlighting crimson, to connote the Harvard connection), a letterhead, and a typeface for our official stationery, and we drafted an announcement. We sent this announcement to every attorney we had ever worked with, heard of, or could find in the Yellow Pages under every imaginable category that might have had some psychiatric component (I believe this excluded only admiralty practice and the law of the sea).

All this effort did *nothing*. We received a few form announcements from two or three firms about *their* offerings, but the net effect for all this time, thought, and expense resembled our own responses to offers that come in the mail to sell us insurance. The result was tantamount to letting a drop of water fall into a large lake. Most recipients almost certainly awarded our announcement the coveted circular file disposition.

The Key Approach

As time went on, it became absolutely clear that only one reliable mechanism among attorneys (and for that matter, clinicians) led to forensic referrals: word of mouth. Support for this theory came from Harvey Research in 1994, which revealed that 77% of attorneys got the names of expert witnesses from other attorneys (that is, word of mouth). Based on this reasoning, an expert's marketing strategy shifts to generating favorable word of mouth. Ordinary advertising in *Lawyers' Weekly,* for example, is suspect and not reliable as an approach (see also Chapter 4 in this volume).

The Delicate Balance

In all approaches to marketing, the expert must strike a delicate balance between honest and reasonable efforts to offer services to potential clients and sleazy, opportunistic commercialized hustling for business—or the *appearance* thereof. The balance must be struck between dualities such as generating word of mouth versus hucksterism, sharing useful information versus being pushy, and pride and confidence in your work versus hired gun certainty. The problem with some forms of getting the word out is that you may not know how a particular listing is regarded within the legal field. Do most attorneys view the names of experts listed in a particular directory as proven hired guns? How could you find out honestly (that is, would you get a straight answer from the attorneys you would want to work for)?

Strategies

Various approaches are recommended as you develop and market your forensic practice: announce, inform, list, speak, write, and unspecialize.

Announce

If the circumstances call for an announcement (which is not common), the announcement should display the professionalism that you plan to bring to the work. Thus, it should be tasteful, informative, and factual. Avoid any hype, including listing services you are not truly expert in. Describe those services you can authentically offer, and send it to attorneys and clinicians, hand it out at a lecture, or use it in some other appropriate way.

Some experts replace the announcement with a minibrochure: a single, trifold sheet of fine paper with a brief description of the expert and the services. It is unclear whether the brochure is superior to the announcement and may be better utilized as the second item of information sent after an initial communication.

Inform

The information about your availability may be directed to four possible audiences: 1) your clinical peer group, 2) your forensic peer group, 3) attorneys, and 4) judges.

For your clinical peers, it is appropriate to let them know in face-to-face or telephone encounters about your new interests in forensic work. Alumni bulletins and class reunions are also opportunities to get the word out.

Although your forensic peers may seem to be your competition, they will be useful to you in several ways. First, they may turn away a case because of a conflict of interest, too little time, previous associations with the attorneys on the other side, or other reasons. If you inform your peer groups about your availability, they may think of you at that point. National meetings of professional associations (such as those of the American Psychiatric Association [APA] and American Academy of Psychiatry and the Law [AAPL]) and local chapters of other organizations offer additional opportunities for informing peers about openings in your caseload.

Attorneys whom you can inform include your own attorney, if you have one, and lawyer neighbors and friends who might pass your name along.

Finally, judges may need your services. If you are moving into a new town, you may wish to send a short, polite letter informing local judges of your availability for forensic services. Serving as a guardian ad litem is an excellent way to meet attorneys and judges who can evaluate your work and spread the word.

List

Listings can be effective as well. Consider listing yourself in your APA district branch's directory as having special interest in forensic work and in the AAPL member directory. Other listings in compendia such as "Attorneys' Guide to Experts" and those of the National Forensic Center may be viewed as less clearly objective and neutral and may pose similar risks to outright advertising; however, these publications may be explored.

Speak

Lecturing on relevant medicolegal or forensic topics is also an introduction to populations who may use your services, such as clinicians and lawyers. Your podium demeanor may convey at least a little about your expected performance on the witness stand.

Do not attempt to schedule yourself for a freestanding lecture on new developments in the insanity defense or whatever; no one will show. Instead, sign up as an entry in an existing lecture series, such as hospital grand rounds, departmental conferences, or established continuing medical education programs.

Become active in your district branch legislative committees and processes. You will be exposed to attorneys and legislators, both of whom may be potential referral sources.

Finally, try to become involved in local media such as call-in shows, which are often seeking a stable of experts to comment on medicolegal stories of the moment. Admittedly, this skill is acquired, and media exposure may open you to crank calls, ambush journalism, and similar humiliations. The APA Public Affairs Office provides some guidance in dealing with the media, but the wounds of experience are probably and ultimately the best teacher.

Write

In our computerized modern age, many referrals to psychiatrists come from publications, the topics of which appear on the screens of attorneys' computer searches. Although it is useful exposure and a valuable resource to write an analysis, review, or commentary and have it published, good visibility also can be obtained by letters to the editor of major journals reporting on a single case or responding to the articles or letters of other contributors.

Unspecialize

For the novice expert, the temptation to specialize from the outset is strong: "In my search to become a media darling and celebrity, I will work only on high-profile, widely publicized mass murders." This is a losing strategy. Begin your career by *un*specializing, wherein you follow the ancient maxim, No case too small. Even minor, trivial cases allow you to be observed in action by potential employers.

The most gratifying outcome is when the attorney for the other side of a case retains you on a later case, based on your fine performance at the deposition.

From the absolute onset of your career, integrity must be your watchword, a point that cannot be overemphasized. It does not matter if the first 3 cases (or 5 or 10) that you get are ones that you must turn down as baseless. It does not matter if the case is trivial or small potatoes. Do not bend the truth to satisfy the attorney; one turn to the Dark Side of the Force, and your course as hired gun may be marked. It may then take you years of work to unblemish your reputation.

In the same vein, your forensic examinations and your first oral and written reports must be meticulous and carefully crafted, no matter how slight the issue. Consider taking on some pro bono work as well, even at the outset. You will derive no income, but you will obtain valuable exposure.

Additional Pointers

The issue may seem trivial, but its importance cannot be overstated: return telephone calls *promptly*. It is astonishing how often prompt telephone responses are ignored as somehow demeaning or conveying inappropriate eagerness, but every attorney whose call you return promptly will greatly appreciate it and be pleasantly surprised. The difficulty of reaching most practitioners is legendary and exceeded only by the problem of getting them to call back. Return telephone calls are the easiest marketing device and one of the most effective.

Remember how your parents tried to impress on you during elementary school the value of thank-you notes? It's still true. Remember to thank your referral sources, including attorneys and fellow clinicians, for referrals. Consider sending a curriculum vitae even to those attorneys whose cases you haven't had the time to review.

Finally, recall the value of brokering. You are saying to the calling attorney, "I can't take this case (because of time, conflict, specific required expertise), but I will take it upon myself to find somebody good who can." Although you are feeding the competition, you are also revealing yourself as a good first stop on the search for a good expert. In analogy with clinical referrals, whereby you would refer someone only to a practitioner whom you would trust treating a member of your family, choose only those experts whom you would be confident to have on your side if you were being sued for something.

Building a practice on word of mouth is slow, at times trying and demanding of patience, but no other method is as reliable, sound, and effective. I reemphasize the point made in Chapter 1 in this book: it is important to have a salaried job and/or a private practice to insulate you from slavery to the fiscal pressures of forensic work.

10

The Expert on the Road

If you take only cases in your immediate neighborhood (such as might happen when you work for a court clinic) or if you are already a seasoned traveler, this chapter will be too obvious and not relevant to your needs. In this chapter, I address some tips and strategies for the expert who is inexperienced in traveling to cases, examinations, or interviews.

The basic situation I describe is one in which you travel by airplane to the city where the trial (or deposition or interview) is being held, stay overnight in a hotel or similar setting, testify or interview the next day, and return that day or the following one. For cases that involve land travel, you may make the appropriate adjustments.

Some General Recommendations

Travel Information

Travel guides are available everywhere, and general information can be obtained from books, travel agents, and your colleagues. I recommend *The Packing Book* (1) as an excellent resource if you always arrive at your travel destination with the wrong clothes in serious disarray and find you have left out several important items. Another useful reference is *Jet Smart* (2). Some experts like to subscribe to an official airline guide for creative problem solving if they are marooned in distant locations because of altered or canceled flights.

I strongly recommend enrolling in a 24-hour travel service with a toll-free number and a separate customer service number. These services can book flights, cars, and hotels directly and save you much time and stress on the telephone.

Leveraging

I also recommend that if you find yourself traveling more than once every 3 months, you enroll in every airline frequent flyer program, every major hotel program, and every major rental car program (note that because of partnerships, some of these programs are clustered so that enrollment in the Marriott program, for example, partners you with several airlines and car rental agencies). These enrollments are especially useful and well worth it in travel emergencies when program members may get the last available room or airplane seat or special assistance.

Also consider using a major credit card that is tied to one of these programs for a "multiplier effect." Among other benefits, this connection permits you to use free travel for the occasional pro bono case you may undertake.

Time Planning and Packing

As noted in Chapter 7 in this volume, you must assume significant time delays and be prepared for your time commitment for court appearances to go into a second or even third day; rarely, the process takes even longer. An effective strategy is to plan on at least a second day and to pack accordingly with a second outfit for court, extra shirts or blouses, underwear, and socks, stockings, or hose. Opt for crushproof fabrics and materials whenever possible. Try on everything before you pack it, especially if you have not worn it for a while, to ensure that it still fits, matches, looks professional, and is in good repair. Consult with significant others for their opinions if needed.

You probably can get away with taking just one wrinkleproof suit or outfit if you guard it with paranoid vigilance, especially in flight, and one pair of shoes, although you may wish to wear sneakers on the airplane and pack the shoes you'll wear to court (medium heels for women; polished shoes for men and women). Sneakers also allow you to sprint through airports to your connecting flight if you are late. If the trial runs longer than a day or so, you may have to use the hotel's laundry and dry-cleaning facilities.

The Ethics of Billing

Bill strictly according to your fee agreement. Consider negotiating a separate travel retainer per fee agreement to cover the time and costs (for example, 1 day at your day rate, because some law firms are slow to reimburse hotel and plane expenses). It is considered appropriate to seek reimbursement from the retaining attorney for the cost of your hotel room or similar accommodation, for one or two telephone calls per day to the office to check on things, for one telephone call to the family, and for the regular three meals but not alcoholic beverages, in-room movies, massages, or 2-hour long-distance calls to your paramour. Separate business from personal comfort; do not bill for sleep (you do it anyway).

My colleagues and I are studying the ethical complexities of billing more than one retaining attorney for trips involving multiple cases. The results are not yet tabulated, so empirical guidance is lacking (the issue of double billing is addressed nowhere in the forensic literature). Until data emerge, a useful principle is to avoid double billing in any form. For example, if you are flying to a case and use air travel time to review the case, do not bill separately for that work because you are already being paid a day rate. If you review a different case on the way back, you may bill for that time but not for the ticket because the first case paid the whole trip already. Seek equitable division of costs for multiple case trips, which are, fortunately, rare but extremely stressful when they do occur.

Secrets of Packing

The Travel Suitcase

Go to any airport, and you will see that most of traveling humanity seems to have caught on to the fact that flight attendants do a heck of a lot of traveling and may know some things we ordinary mortals don't, such as the value of the roll-along suitcase. This fantastic invention is a small, usually black, rectangular suitcase with a handle extended upward on two metal tubes, permitting the suitcase to be rolled along behind you like a tiny rickshaw. This device is the traveling expert's best friend. A briefcase often is sold with this suitcase and can be snapped or hooked piggyback onto the suitcase. It is possible, then, to pack for 2 or 3 days of travel and bring most of the key documents in a case along for review while remaining in full carry-on mode. (Avoid checking baggage if you can. You have enough to worry about without having your materials for the case in Chicago while you are in Cleveland.) In addition, these roll-alongs often fit either in the overhead compartment or, with a little applied topology, even under the seat in some cases.

Some of these roll-along suitcases include a special compartment so that a suit can be folded and carried along inside. It is not clear if the bag keeps the outfit suitably wrinkle free as advertised, but you may wish to experiment with a friend's suitcase. Alternatively, you may opt to wear the suit or outfit and guard it.

Do not skimp or economize on a roll-along suitcase. Examine your purchase closely for multiple pockets and compartments (good for a thin, compact plastic raincoat or poncho). Buy a durable, well-made suitcase by Travelpro, Sharper Image, Samsonite, or other reputable company. Keep in mind that being able to fit the suitcase under the seat is a distinct advantage, an advantage you lose if it is too bulky or bulges when packed.

The Kit

Whether you call it a travel kit, Dopp kit, makeup bag, or toiletries case, it is indispensable to your successful travel ventures. If you do a lot of traveling, I recommend having it prepacked with duplicate goods rather than trying to fill it each time from your daily cosmetics and such. The kit must have a waterproof liner of plastic or nylon; cloth or even ballistic nylon fabric, a popular material, will leak thin liquids such as cologne, mouthwash, or after-shave. Remember that pressurized cans can blow up during air travel (rare, but it does happen); sticks, creams, squeeze bottles, or pump canisters are good alternatives.

In psychoanalytic theory, the principle of multiple function is one of the basics of a dynamic understanding of mental life. It is definitely a basic principle for assembling your kit. What you take should have similar versatility.

Remember also that your kit should contain items that permit repair, remedy, and cleaning. These should include sewing items, such as a variety of buttons and threads to match your clothes; stain-remover sticks that do not contain toxic petrochemicals; safety pins in various sizes; extra shoelaces; and rubber bands, tape, and string.

A small, multifunction "pharmacy" also should be included. It should contain not only your usual prescription medications but also emergency supplies such as headache remedies, antacids, decongestants, and similar medications. Antihistamine tablets and an antihistamine or steroid cream will be useful for unexpected allergic reactions.

Miscellaneous Items

Consider taking along a lightweight workout outfit if that is part of your routine. Wear your workout or running shoes on the plane, and pack the rest of the gear. A pair of nylon running-type shorts and a quick-drying top are versatile items that can be worn not only for exercise but also in the Jacuzzi or in your hotel room as a comfortable lounging outfit while you review the case.

Other useful miscellaneous items include scissors and tweezers in protective sheaths; adhesive bandages of various sizes and types; a small, light flashlight for power outages and searching under beds for lost items; extra eyeglasses or contacts if you wear them; eyeglass screwdrivers and replacement screws; extra combs; and a miniature tool kit, such as a Swiss army knife or the various compact versions now on the market.

If you travel with a laptop computer, remember to carry light extension cords and voltage adapters, as well as extra diskettes and the instruction manual. A cellular telephone is extremely useful to reach your attorney's office from out-of-the-way places, to alter travel plans, to check messages, and so forth. The telephones at airports are often mobbed, especially when you need them most (such as when there are flight changes).

Emergency Items

Neurotic fears can certainly flower when you travel, but some precautions seem sensible. Besides a small flashlight, I carry a compact "smoke hood," a device that comes in a packet or canister and that is placed over the head in the event of a hotel fire. You breathe through a filter that lasts long enough, in theory, for you to get out of the toxic smoke and gases to safety. This item is available through a number of catalogs.

Almost all modern hotels in the United States have smoke detectors, but you can buy your own compact version, often hooked to a travel alarm clock. This latter item also is probably quite vital as a backup for the wake-up system used by the hotel (which rarely, although occasionally, fails).

Secrets of Flying

Consider upgrading to first class to allow you to spread out the case materials for in-flight review. Drink water steadily to avoid travel dehydration; on very dry flights, try breathing through a moistened towel for short periods. A decongestant before flight may be helpful if you are the least bit stuffy or have a cold.

Seriously consider avoiding airline food entirely, or order special low-fat meals. Some experts nibble an "energy bar" during flight and postpone having lunch or dinner until they reach their destination. If you do eat on the plane, ignore manners or inhibitions and use your napkin like a lobster bib, tucked in at or near the chin and spread across your front, to protect your clothes from the effects of turbulence or maladroit flight attendants. If you have a disability, call the airline early to check on facilities, procedures, and special arrangements.

Secrets of Staying

If you are unfamiliar with the expert art of "fly in, testify, fly out," this discussion will be helpful; experienced travelers can skip this discussion.

The traveling expert is sometimes torn between staying at a cold, institutional hotel or motel and cadging free lodging with friends or relatives in the area. The latter appears at first glance both socially desirable and economical, because someone is paying your way to the location.

I recommend the hotel or motel for several reasons. First, you are undistracted by social obligations and family strife or background noise. Second, it is more professional to meet with your attorney the night before the trial in a hotel room or conference room; this is, after all, a business trip. After the trial, of course, you are free to visit friends and family at your own discretion.

My first move on entering a hotel room, after I put down my luggage, is to make a beeline for the hotel's alarm clock or clock radio. This move ensures that some eager-beaver salesperson who had to rise at 4:00 A.M. did not leave the clock set to that time so that you wake before dawn to the snarl of the alarm in a full-fledged panic attack and cannot go back to sleep, rendering you bleary-eyed and incoherent on the stand the next day and giving rise to unfounded rumors about your substance abuse.

My second move often is to arrange a do-it-yourself humidification of the room. Whether the room's air system is heating in winter or cooling in summer, the air is invariably dry in most hotels, a situation that can leave you hoarse, congested, and headachy on the stand. A simple but highly effective method is to soak a washcloth or hand towel in cold water, wring it out thoroughly so that it doesn't drip, and fasten it over the air inlet in your room so that the incoming air blows through the damp cloth (this may entail *carefully* standing on a chair if the inlet is near the ceiling). If a paper clip or safety pin does not suspend the cloth or towel well, you can often wad up the corners and jam them between the top louvers of the inlet so that the cloth or towel hangs across the incoming air inlet. Remoisten it as needed. Don't forget to set the room thermostat to your accustomed household temperature.

Hang up everything and spray items that need it with commercially available wrinkle-smoothing liquid, or hang clothes from the shower rod over a tub of hot water so that the "sauna effect" steams clothes smooth. Some, but not all, hotels provide irons.

Arrange your wake-up call so that it allows ample time for an unrushed breakfast and last-minute case review; back up the call with your travel alarm. Finding a hotel that is close to the courthouse saves you much last-minute rushing and buys you some morning time as well. Traveling to the courthouse with your attorney may provide a valuable opportunity to be updated on the case and to get in touch with the emotional tone of the courtroom and the proceedings to this point, an essential part of effective testimony.

Secrets of Eating

In traveling to court, obviously you should eat lightly and stick to what is familiar to you. Experimenting with culinary exotica is asking for a case of turista at worst; nausea on the witness stand also may be misinterpreted. It is probably safest to avoid all alcohol during the trip before testimony; have your martini on the airplane home after it is all over.

At court during the lunch break, also eat lightly. Consider only coffee or iced tea or a fruit drink to avoid afternoon sluggishness of thought and energy level. After court, you can have a serious meal without ill effect.

Secrets of Sleeping

One of the greatest pitfalls for the traveling expert is dealing with the stress of sleeping in a different place, or even a different time zone, by using either alcohol or sleeping pills (barbiturates or benzodiazepines) at bedtime. These have ill effects, including hangovers, and with sleeping pills, actual memory loss can occur—the last thing you need. Far better results accrue from sleep hygiene maneuvers, hot baths, breathing techniques, and similar relaxants. Melatonin in low doses (about 1 mg) appears to be reasonably effective without ill effects, but all the data are not in. When possible, of course, plan your trip to allow time for recovery from jet lag.

Many travelers find it helpful to block out morning sunlight with the drapes, either by closing them completely or fastening gaping fabrics with safety pins.

A useful approach to dealing with the problem of ambient noise (such as the flushing of the toilet next door at 4:00 A.M., the roar of early morning delivery or garbage trucks in the hotel parking lot or airplanes overhead, the chatter of housekeeping staff just outside your door) is *white noise.* This term refers to sounds containing all frequencies, just as white light contains all color wavelengths. Ordinary AM radio static and the sound of surf are two examples of white noise. Setting the radio to a "nonstation" to generate static and the television to a "nonchannel" to get the sound that usually accompanies snow on the television screen (modern digital televisions usually do not permit this) are both methods of achieving this end. Catalogs sell portable battery-operated white-noise generators. White noise masks ambient noise effectively and creates a sensory monotony that is a significant sleep aid, without aftereffects; I recommend it.

What to Take to Court

Courthouses are notably lacking in amenities, so you may have to carry some supplies in your pocket or purse. Examples include prescription medications that you need during the course of a long day; some alcohol wipes or other pocket-size cleansing products for hand cleaning, stain removal, or refreshment; cough drops, mints, or throat lozenges; and a headache remedy for the obvious problem. Note that anything in a metal pillbox or foil-wrapped packet may set off the sensitive metal detectors used in some courthouses.

Although some of the pointers in this chapter probably state the obvious, I hope that these tips make your travel easier and less surprising. I welcome your suggestions and favorite travel tips.

References

1. Gilford J: The Packing Book: Secrets of the Carry-On Traveler. Berkeley, CA, Ten Speed Press, 1994 (An excellent guide to what to take and how to pack it; sample wardrobes and general travel pointers included as well.)
2. Fairechild D: Jet Smart: Over 200 Tips for Beating Jet Lag. Berkeley, CA, Celestial Arts Publishing, 1992 (A bit New Age but filled with useful tips from a former flight attendant who really knows the ropes.)

11

Epilogue

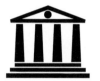

I hope this introduction to the challenging yet always fascinating role of expert witness has been instructive and helpful to you, not only in performing your task successfully but also in helping you avoid some of the pitfalls of beginning a new career sideline.

Although some forces in society, including our medical colleagues, decry the expert witness function and voice arguments for its abolition, the courts will continue, from all evidence, to require our services. The better we are at meeting the courts' needs with ethical, effective, and helpful testimony, the more we serve this valuable and necessary function.

If I have made too many assumptions about you, the reader, or have taken too much for granted about your background and experience in any portion of this text, consider first reading the companion volume, *The Psychiatrist in Court: A Survival Guide*. That book may fill in some of the blanks.

As always, I welcome comments and suggestions from readers to correct, expand, or render this text more useful.

APPENDIX 1

Standard Fee Agreement

This example of a standard fee agreement is annotated by lowercase letters in parentheses (annotations are explained at the end of the text for this agreement). Each detail in this agreement emerged from an attempt at evasion of fiscal responsibility by some attorney or insurer.

Thomas G. Gutheil, M.D.
Standard Letter of Agreement

1. In consideration of his agreeing (a) to serve as consultant/expert (b) to the undersigned, Dr. Gutheil shall be reimbursed for all time spent on the case, including portal-to-portal local travel (c), at a rate of $_____ per hour plus expenses.
2. For out-of-state travel, the rate of payment shall be $_____per day and $_____ per half-day (4 hours or fraction thereof) plus all expenses, including travel by first-class conveyance and appropriate lodging if needed. Before such travel is undertaken, a retainer of $_____ specific to this travel is expected (d). Please note that because of vacation scheduling, Dr. Gutheil will be unavailable for testimony in person during the month of August (e).
3. Payment in a timely (f) manner, made out to Dr. Gutheil by name (g), is the sole responsibility of the retaining attorney or insurer (h), irrespective of case outcome (i). Overdue accounts may accrue interest at 6% per annum, prorated (j). Failure to comply may void this agreement (k), leaving the retaining attorney or insurer individually liable for any unpaid balance (l). Dr. Gutheil's FID# is _____.

4. A nonrefundable retainer (m) of $_____ is required before commencement of work on the case, as an advance against which expenses are billed (n).

5. Signature below indicates agreement with all (o) these terms; please return one copy to Dr. Gutheil.

Signed,

_____   _____
Attorney or Firm Representative (p)   Date

Note: Please send all case materials to (address)

Annotations

(a) "Consideration" and "agreeing" are trigger words that signal to attorneys, based on their training, that this is a formal contract.

(b) You are initially retained as a consultant; whether you become an expert depends on your taking the case as meritorious and the attorney's accepting you as an expert witness (for deposition and/or trial).

(c) To cut through nit-picking, the "clock" starts when you leave your home or office for court and stops when you return to office or home, thus, "portal-to-portal."

(d) For unexplained reasons, attorneys are sometimes slow to reimburse travel expenses for interview, deposition, or trial travel. Because you will be investing a fair amount in the travel costs, I recommend asking for this secondary retainer before travel.

(e) If you know when your vacation is, it saves everyone time and heartache if you spell it out. This information frees up the attorney to ask for continuance or rescheduling, take a videotaped deposition, or even retain another expert.

(f) You have the right to request timely payment to prevent excessive back balance buildup. If the retaining party is relentlessly slow, you may decide to withdraw.

(g) If you are the sole proprietor, or a member of a corporation or group practice, make that clear so that you don't waste a lot of time swapping checks between payees.

(h) Some attorneys, dunned for appropriately earned fees, will throw up their hands in mock exasperation and say, "You're right, Doc, but what can I do? That client just won't honor his or her obligations." Make it clear that you do not work for the client and that the attorney or insurer (in some civil defense cases) is the responsible party. Working for the client, moreover, can constitute a bias.

(i) Your fee is, as it ethically should be, noncontingent. A case decision that goes against the side retaining you is not grounds for nonpayment.

(j) This is a standard rate of interest on overdue accounts and an incentive for timely payment.

(k) You must be free to withdraw from the case if the contract is breached; this statement makes the attorney agree to that possibility.

(l) If you do withdraw, that does not mean you should not be paid for the work already done; this clause makes that explicit.

(m) On rare occasions, attorneys may attempt to tie up (legally bind) an expert by retaining him or her on paper to prevent the other side from consulting him or her. Such attorneys may pay the retainer, making you ineligible for participation with the other side; give you no work to do; and, after settling the case, ask for their retainer back, because you did no work. You have been sandbagged, at no cost to the attorney but at lost time and possible income to you. Making the retainer nonrefundable tends to eliminate such shenanigans.

(n) The retainer is not only a means of establishing the contract but also an actual advance against expenses. When this retainer is depleted, some experts simply submit additional invoices; others ask for a second retainer (see also Appendix 2 in this volume).

(o) "All" is a small word but one that prevents attorneys from selecting only some terms to agree with.

(p) You are agreeing to accept signature from a different attorney or a paralegal, for example, if the attorney is out of the country; this does not weaken the contractual ties.

APPENDIX 2

Detailed Fee Agreement

The following is an example of a colleague's more detailed fee agreement.

LARRY H. STRASBURGER, M.D.
Clinical and Forensic Psychiatry
(Address)
(Date)
Re: (Case)

Dear (Attorney):

This will confirm our agreement regarding my providing psychiatric consulting services with regard to the above-referenced matter. I will charge an hourly rate of $_____ with an initial retainer of $_____ due upon execution of this letter of agreement. This retainer will constitute a credit balance until exhausted. Thereafter, if it appears that substantial services are yet to be rendered, I may require an additional retainer. Any credit balance remaining will be refunded upon the termination of my services. It is understood and agreed that timely payment for my service and expenses will be solely the responsibility of the attorney, and is in no way contingent upon the outcome of any litigation or settlement.

Used with permission.

Psychiatric services may include an initial consultation, psychiatric interview or evaluation, interviews with family members or other persons, consultation with counsel, review of records, and report preparation. If travel from my office is necessary to perform any of these services, the hourly rates will apply to portal-to-portal travel time, and all travel expenses will be reimbursed. All travel shall be by first-class conveyance. Missed appointments by clients or attorneys will be charged for unless 48-hour notice of cancellation is given. It is understood and agreed that you will pay all out-of-pocket expenses in connection with this matter, including secretarial service, postage, literature research, photocopying, long-distance telephone calls, messenger services, etc.

It is further understood and agreed that should a decision be made to call me as a witness at any deposition or court proceeding, compensation for my time in giving testimony shall be as follows: I shall be compensated at the rate of $_____ per half-day (4 hours or any part thereof) or $_____ per full day (in excess of 4 hours). For depositions and court appearances requiring travel beyond the Boston area I shall be compensated at the rate of $_____ per calendar day plus all expenses. Time spent in preparing for testimony shall be billed at the hourly rate specified above. I shall be given 2 weeks' notice of deposition or trial in order to make adequate preparation. There shall be on deposit with me a retainer in the amount of $_____ 5 working days prior to commencement of testimony. If notification of cancellation is made less than 2 working days before the scheduled deposition or trial, no refund of the retainer deposit will be made.

It is further understood and agreed that failure of any other party or counsel in any litigation to pay expenses or witness fees, expert or otherwise, as prescribed by statute, court rule, court order or agreement shall not relieve your obligation to pay my fees and expenses for time spent in testifying or preparing to testify. Nor shall such failure relieve your obligation to have on deposit, prior to my testimony, the retainer discussed above.

I will send you a monthly statement, setting forth the nature of the services rendered since the prior billing, along with a listing of out-of-pocket expenses. Any excess over the retainer balance is due upon receipt.

If the foregoing fee basis meets with your approval, please so indicate by signing this letter and returning it to me with your check for the retainer. Please keep a copy of this letter for your records.

Sincerely,

Larry H. Strasburger, M.D.
Diplomate, American Board of Psychiatry and Neurology
Diplomate, American Board of Forensic Psychiatry
AGREED AS TO FEE AND EXPENSE BASIS:

Attorney Signature and Date:

_____

APPENDIX 3

Suggested Readings

Note that many of the following suggested readings cover the expert witness's role in general fields, not just psychiatry. All, however, provide information useful for the psychiatric expert. These sources are meant to supplement those provided at the ends of the chapters in this book, as well as those found in the companion volume, *The Psychiatrist in Court: A Survival Guide.*

Babitsky S, Mangraviti JJ: How to Excel During Cross Examination: Techniques for Experts That Work. Falmouth, MA, SEAK, 1997

Brodsky SL: Testifying in Court: Guidelines and Maxims for the Expert Witness. Washington, DC, American Psychological Association, 1991

Clifford RC: Qualifying and Attacking Expert Witnesses. Santa Ana, CA, James Publishing, 1993

Dorram PB: The Expert Witness. Chicago, IL, The American Planning Association, 1982

Feder HA: Succeeding as an Expert Witness. Glenwood Springs, CO, Tageh Press, 1993

Isele WP: Under Oath: Tips for Testifying. Horsham, PA, LRP Publications, 1995

McHale MJ, Covise LL, Mulligan WG, et al: Expert Witnesses: Direct and Cross Examination. New York, Wiley Law Publications, 1997

O'Barr WM: Linguistic Evidence: Language, Power and Strategy in the Courtroom. San Diego, CA, Academic Press, 1982

Poynter D: The Expert Witness Handbook: Tips and Techniques for the Litigation Consultant. Santa Barbara, CA, Para Publishing, 1987

Quen JM: The Psychiatrist in the Courtroom: Selected Papers of Bernard L. Diamond. Hillsdale, NJ, Analytic Press, 1994

Rabinoff MA, Holmes SP: The Forensic Expert's Guide to Litigation: the Anatomy of a Lawsuit. Danvers, MA, LRP Publications, 1996

Veitch TH: The Consultant's Guide to Litigation Services: How to Be an Expert Witness. New York, Wiley, 1993

Younger I: The Art of Cross Examination. Washington, DC, American Bar Association, Section of Litigation, 1976

Zobel HB, Rons SN: Doctors and the Law: Defendants and Expert Witnesses. New York, WW Norton, 1993

Index